The Yoga Healing Bible

The Yoga
Healing Bible

Find the best postures, meditations, relaxations,
and breathing exercises for complete
physical and spiritual balance

Sally Parkes

CHARTWELL
BOOKS, INC.

A QUANTUM BOOK

This edition published in 2013 by
CHARTWELL BOOKS, INC.
A division of BOOK SALES INC.,
276 Fifth Avenue, Suite 206
New York, New York 10001
USA

Copyright © 2013 Quantum Publishing Ltd

ISBN 13: 978-0-7858-3065-8

Produced by
Quantum Publishing Ltd
The Old Brewery
6 Blundell Street
London N7 9BH

QUMTYHB

Assistant Editor: Jo Morley
Editors: Hazel Eriksson and Sam Kennedy
Consultant Editor: Sally Parkes
Production Manager: Rohana Yusof
Publisher: Sarah Bloxham

Packaged by Guy Croton
Publishing Services, Tonbridge, Kent

Quantum would like to thank and
acknowledge the following for supplying the
pictures reproduced in this book:

Guy Croton: pp 10, 14, 22, 23, 38, 39, 40,
41, 177, 193
iStock: pp 11, 16, 11, 171, 175, 181, 200
stock.xchng: pp 13, 15, 173, 178, 184, 187,
195, 196

All other photographs and illustrations are
the copyright of Quantum Publishing Ltd

While every effort has been made to
credit contributors, Quantum would like
to apologize should there have been any
omissions or errors.

Some of the material in this book originally
appeared in *Simple Yoga Techniques* and
Yoga Made Easy.

Printed in China by Midas Printing
International Ltd.

Contents

Foreword

In the western hemisphere yoga has become a very popular form of physical exercise, and it is easy to think that yoga is only about twisting and stretching the body, breathing practices, and a little chanting here and there. However, these are simply tools to assist us on our path to still the mind.

The ancient sage Pantanjali said:

"Yoga citta vrtti nirodhaha."
"The restraint of the modifications of the mind-stuff is yoga."

This quote tells us that practices of asana, pranayama, chanting, and kriyas (cleansing techniques) are ultimately stepping stones for reaching a point where we can control our mind-stuff, our thoughts. That is the ultimate goal of practicing yoga. It is very beneficial for us to become physically and mentally stronger, more flexible and of clearer thought, but if the mind is still constantly busy and unsettled, there is still work to do.

For the last twenty years, yoga and other traditions rooted in spirituality have always been of interest to me. I always felt there must be more to life and I just couldn't buy into the idea of a "set life plan and then you die" idea—it just didn't make sense to me. I knew there was another path for me. I had always enjoyed regular exercise and loved the high it gave me, as I often found I felt the most relaxed mentally during my long distance running or cycling sessions. I would find the chatter of my mind would begin to quiet and I felt totally inspired and happy, but several injuries soon made me realize that this path was not sustainable on a long-term basis.

I had already enjoyed one of my first yoga books, *Moving into Stillness* by Erich Schiffman, when I started to attend Iyengar yoga classes. I found the classes very challenging and so I was totally engaged mentally. Over the first two years of regular Iyengar yoga practice, all my injuries healed themselves and my body became pain free. I was a yoga convert!

At that time, I was reading a lot of texts by A. C. Bhaktivedanta Swami Prabhupada of the Krishna Consciousness Yoga System. The more I read, the more I realized that I began to understand the philosophy of yoga and it was thanks to such texts and the Yoga Sutras that I finally discovered what yoga was actually all about; it is a journey through the Eight Limbs, a yoga system that gives us tools to keep climbing the yogic ladder and allows us to deal with whatever is thrown at us more effectively. The fluctuations of our mental stillness gradually become less and less as we become less reactive.

It is when mental stillness is attained, that yoga begins to filter through to our thoughts, words, and deeds, and we can truly embrace its philosophy. We start to see The Eight Limbs with new eyes and our journey into yoga begins to come to life, as it reaches all corners of our life.

And so with this in mind, I feel that The Yoga Healing Bible is an invaluable guide to your journey into yoga. The asanas have been carefully compiled into an order that will gradually strengthen and open the body and balance the nervous system. There is emphasis on correct breathing and relaxation, which are paramount to an effective yoga practice. All these elements lead to a well rounded yoga practice and are as important as one another, and are greater than their sum.

The practice of yoga makes your world shine a little more, and you begin to treat yourself and others with more kindness, you are more at ease in your body, and the continuous chatter of your thoughts starts, little by little, to become more quiet. I hope you enjoy your journey into stillness.

Sally Parkes
Consultant Editor

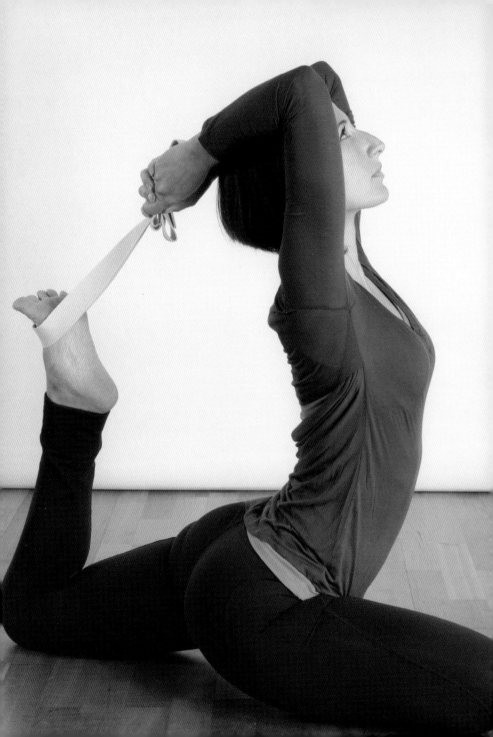

An Introduction to Yoga

Today, you can travel all over the place and find a yoga class in the nearest city or even in your local town. The class may include women and men of various ages, people of various shapes, sizes, and degrees of fitness. It is a discipline and form of exercise that appeals to many different kinds of people, because in our fast-paced, stressful world it offers an accessible and enjoyable means of escape to personal serenity, balance, and contentment. Welcome to the wonderful world of yoga.

Introduction

To the question, "why should an ancient Eastern concept attract millions of practitioners at the beginning of the 21st century?," there is only one answer: because it works.

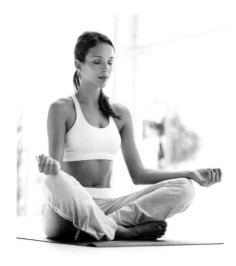

Above Relaxation, a sense of inner peace, contentment, and physical fitness. All of these and many more are the wonderful benefits of yoga.

Yoga offers an attitude to life from which a variety of practices have developed. First and foremost, yoga produces a feeling of peace, both in mind and body. In turn, this feeling stimulates both thought and actions, reminding us of the Latin tag: "Mens sana in corpore sano" ("A healthy mind in a healthy body.")

The word "yoga" means unity or oneness —in other words, a feeling of being part of something. Yoga is one of the original concepts which today would be labeled as holistic. That means the body is related to the breath; both are related to the brain; in turn this links with the mind, which is a part of consciousness. The spelling of holistic, too, is a reminder that the word "whole" is derived from "holy" and therefore you cannot be a "whole" person unless you have a "whole" outlook on life itself.

It is not hard to realize that many of our ills today come from a feeling of isolation—my problems, my pains—a feeling that we are different and separated from others. In the last 50 years there has been a dramatic growth in the understanding of the universal problem now termed "unrelieved stress." At the core of such stress is the sense of fighting a lone battle against great, often insuperable, odds. Today, thousands of doctors who know little or nothing about yoga nevertheless recommend that patients go to yoga classes to help them overcome a variety of stress-related problems. As more research is carried out, so the value of yoga becomes clearer.

Linking Body and Mind

Countless exercising plans are available today. New ones come into fashion and then fade. Almost all of these depend exclusively upon working the body, quite unrelated to the conscious, thinking human being. It would be wrong to say such plans are useless, but their value is limited, because they ignore the proven fact that the mind has a remarkable effect upon the body. Some people quite literally worry themselves to death; while others show a remarkable physical resilience simply because they remain calm and positive. As Buddha declared, some 2,500 years ago, "You are what you think."

The aim of this book is to bring together, as simply as possible, the elements which make up life, so that, without making any undue demands, you can find body, breath, brain, and mind working as one. It sounds difficult, but because it is a natural process, it is really quite simple once you understand what is happening.

The importance of being able to let go and relax in a world with increasing stress factors has become more and more obvious. Medical research showing the value of yoga relaxation techniques in reversing long-held symptoms of high blood pressure, has added a new dimension to the approach of yoga. In recent years, doctors have demonstrated that a yoga-oriented program, involving a change in lifestyle, can actually reverse symptoms of heart disease within 12 months. Through these and other important examples, it has become apparent that there is far more to yoga than performing a number of exercises slowly.

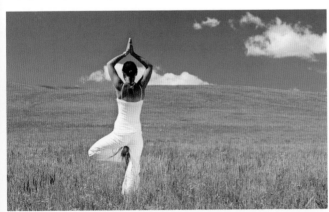

Left Yoga can improve your mental health as well as benefiting you physically, and few pursuits are as successful in uniting the mind and body.

11

How to Use This Book

This is essentially a practical book, although it can be read or browsed for interest. It is designed for beginners and is intended, ideally, as a companion to yoga class attendance.

Opposite Yoga is an incredibly flexible discipline that can be practiced just about anywhere with minimal equipment.

The majority of the contents of this book are devoted to basic instructions for the principal postures of yoga. For each posture, a brief introduction normally leads on to step-by-step directions for performing it correctly. Frequently, these are accompanied by safety advice and/or suggested modifications/adaptations for achieving the posture if the full posture is inappropriate or too difficult. These adaptations often involve the use of simple equipment. Before starting to try to do a pose, be sure to read all the instructions and cautions. (Don't try to peer at the page in an awkward position while trying to perform the posture!) The timings that are given are a guide, but may often be increased as you gain strength and ability in the pose.

The postures are mostly grouped according to how the body relates to the ground: standing, sitting, or lying, and upside-down poses. There is also a section concentrating on relaxation and mental aspects of yoga, and a section presenting more advanced postures, which should not be done without the help of a teacher.

The order in which the postures appear in the book is not the same as the order in which they should be practiced, nor even necessarily the best order in which to learn them. The final section is where the reader learns to put the postures together in order. It offers several ordered practice routines, presented as a progressive course. You may have to make small modifications to these routines and should take health and safety considerations seriously.

Yoga can be a physically demanding discipline and it is important to be aware of your level of fitness and basic physical capacity before embarking on some of the postures demonstrated in this book. If in doubt, consult your doctor before attempting the various poses.

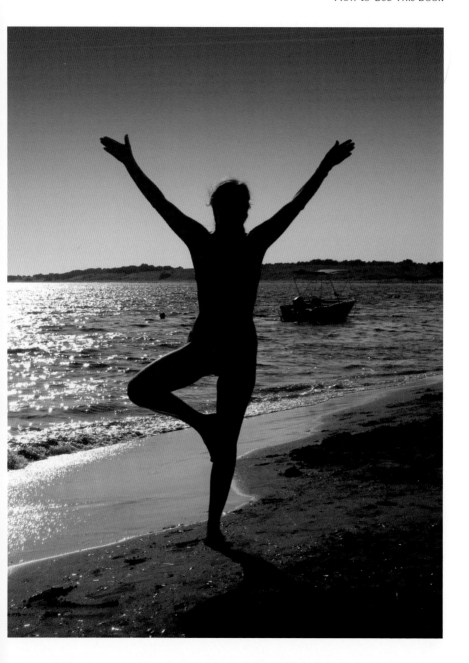

The Origins of Yoga

In India, where yoga was born more than 2,000 years ago, the traditional disciplines survive alongside more modern or Western approaches. This ancient art continues to evolve worldwide.

Below For centuries practitioners of yoga have used meditation, mantras, and breathing techniques to enhance their state of self-awareness.

O ver the centuries, as its influence has spread, yoga has been valued as a discipline that contributes to physical health, psychological wellbeing, and spiritual development. It is a practical philosophy that has proved adaptable to a multitude of cultures and countries, perhaps because it is based on an understanding of our common humanity, rather than the differences that can divide us.

In the Bhagavad Gita—possibly the best-known text of ancient Indian literature—yoga is described as a means of deliverance from pain and sorrow. Suffering is not confined to an era or place, so yoga is just as applicable in any part of the world today as it was in India two millennia ago. It continues to alleviate worldly cares for millions of people.

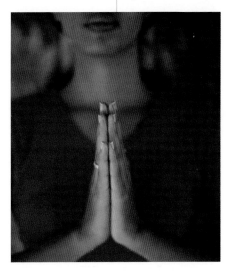

There is a variety of approaches to the goals of yoga, and each may suit different people—some following a devotional path, some seeking realization through knowledge, some through dutiful action. The path that emphasizes control of the mind is called Raja ("kingly") or Hatha yoga. The Sanskrit word "hatha" translates as "force" or "effort;" and it is composed of the words for sun and moon, so that it suggests the balance of complementary influences.

The Sanskrit letter "Om" carries profound meaning for yoga practitioners. By itself or as part of a longer sequence, it constitutes a mantra, a phrase that acts as a focus for meditation. The shape and sound

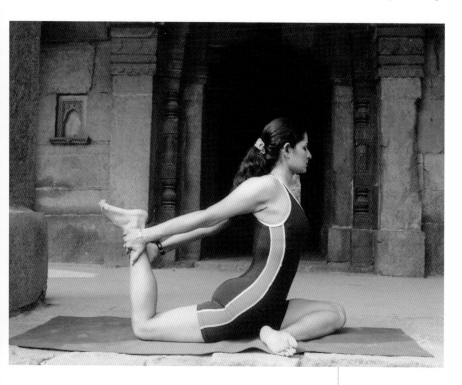

of the syllable symbolize an individual's passage from everyday consciousness to a transcendental state.

Many people think of yoga as the practice of physical exercises requiring flexibility, strength, and balance. Many also know that it includes deep breathing, relaxation, and meditation. These are important aspects of Hatha yoga, although they do not tell the whole story. The desire for better health or easier relaxation is often why people turn to yoga in the first place, and it is not necessary to study Sanskrit or Indian philosophy to reap the rewards of yoga practice. The postures are a means of improving your health; whether you then use your fitter body to carry you along a spiritual path, or simply for greater enjoyment of work and leisure, is up to you. Breathing and relaxation techniques offer you the mental control that is needed for meditation, but you may only want the health benefits and freedom from stress that they offer.

Above Yoga is as popular and as widely practiced in India today as it was more than 2,000 years ago.

15

The Philosophy of Yoga

The word "yoga" carries the meaning of joining or yoking, and so signifies the integration of all parts of the human being—harmony at every level. You can apply harmony to your own life through yoga.

Below and opposite
Follow the lessons of yoga and a sense of "oneness" with the world can soon become yours. The philosophy of yoga has evolved over hundreds of years and has changed countless people's lives for the better.

Accalarding to the classical Indian philosophy of yoga, it is the path to ultimate liberation, by union of the whole being with the Universal Spirit. The words still used to name the yoga postures and the concepts of its philosophy are in Sanskrit, an ancient Indo-European language that is rich in symbolism. In addition to the living tradition of yoga practiced and taught by people of many nationalities, Indian literature provides numerous relevant stories and teachings. In the Yoga Sutras, written by the sage Patanjali (c. 200 B.C.), yoga is said to be the method of calming the restlessness of the conscious mind and of constructively controlling mental and physical energy. Patanjali describes eight limbs (stages) of yoga, a series of steps toward purification of the mind and, ultimately, enlightenment.

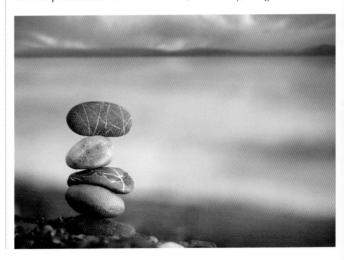

16

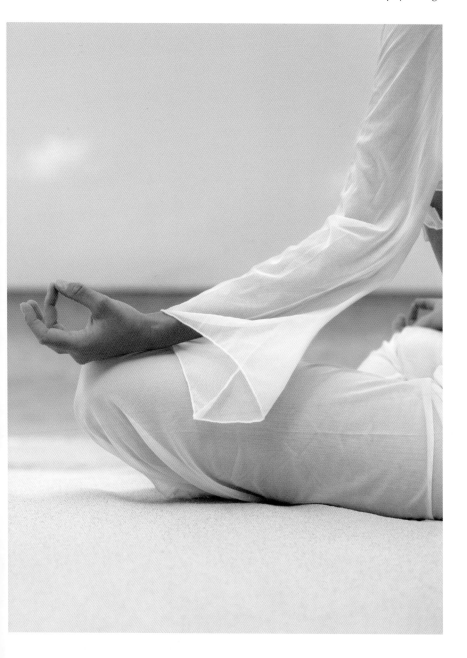

The Eight Stages (Limbs) of Yoga

Limb	Content	Precepts
Yama	Learning to observe the five ethical precepts	Loving non-violence; Honesty; Non-stealing; Self-restraint; Non-acquisitiveness
Niyama	Learning to observe the five guidelines for conduct	Purity; Contentment; Self-discipline; Self-education; Dedication to God
Asana	Practice of postures to strengthen and refine the body and mind	
Pranayama	Controlled breathing (and hence, control of life energy)	
Pratyahara	Freedom from domination by the senses, non-attachment	
Dharana	Concentration, one-pointed mental absorption	
Dhyana	Meditation	
Samadhi	An indescribably blissful state of superconsciousness	

More On Yamas and Niyamas

Yamas are moral restraints, they govern right action, the way we treat others, but also the way we treat ourselves.

1 Ahimsa. Non-harm or Non-violence. This can be thought of as compassion for all living beings, not causing physical or emotional harm. It is important that you also apply this to your own body, especially during yoga practice.

2 Satya. Truth. This is being true to yourself and others and governs open communication. You might want to consider where you stand on certain issues and then be true to that belief in your choices.

3 Asteya. Non-stealing. This covers the traditional sense of not taking something physical that is not yours, but also not taking ideas or behaving in a way that would diminish someone else's life.

4 Bramacharya. This is often described as total celibacy, but realistically governs healthy sexual choices such as choosing partners carefully and having sex from a place of love and mutual respect rather than giving in to the physical desires of the body.

5 Aparigraha. Non-grasping or greedlessness. This means not taking too much, be it food, possessions, or other people's time and energy. This precept teaches us about balance and moderation.

Niyamas are duties or obligations prescribed by a yogi or guru.

1 Saucha. Purity, cleanliness. Of both your physical and mental environment. This extends to the spaces you live and work in and the people you surround yourself with.

2 Santosha. Happiness, contentment. This can be seen as an acceptance of where we are today, in the present moment.

3 Tapas. Self-discipline. This might be a commitment to get on your yoga mat every day, even if it is only for five minutes.

4 Swadhyaya. Self-study. This can also be seen as consciousness or mindfulness. Always question and keep on questioning.

5 Ishvarapranidhana. Devotion. The yoga sutras don't mention a particular god and in that sense yoga is a secular practice. But following the yoga path implies an inherent acceptance of a higher nature or energy, a universal consciousness, a belief in the soul. It doesn't matter what word or image works for you; find something that fits and then commit to it.

19

Equipment and Clothing

There are few requirements for practicing yoga. Clothing should not constrict the movement of the body. Light exercise outfits, such as leggings, vests, and shorts are all suitable.

- For standing poses, use a firm, flat, non-slip surface—a yoga mat is helpful if you tend to slide on the floor.
- In sitting or lying postures, a blanket can protect you from the hardness of the floor, but do not choose one so soft that you sink into it.
- In positions where the feet are wide apart, it can help to press the outer edge of the back foot against the base of a wall. A wall can also help with balance and alignment. Having it at your back while you complete a pose gives you support and lets you know whether you are straight.

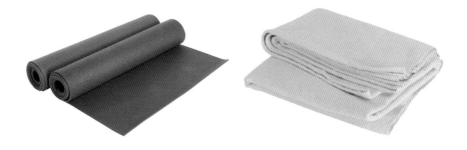

Non-slip mats   Blankets

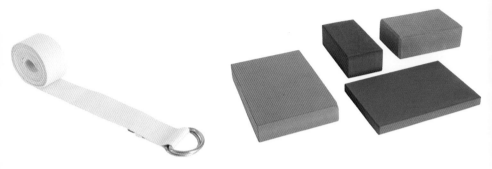

Long belt   Foam blocks

- It is better to place your hand on a chair, block, or brick in a downward-stretching standing pose than to struggle to reach the floor. Trying to go too far can result in injury or strain and distort the shape of the pose.
- In sitting forward bends, avoid strain and distortion by using a long belt, scarf, or similar item to loop around the part that you are trying to reach—usually your foot.
- When sitting, it may be a struggle to successfully straighten the spine. This is often easier if you raise your hips on a firm foam block or some folded blankets.
- Other postures may need similar padding to lift and support a part of the body. For a sturdy support, you may be able to use a thick book or two or more firm foam blocks. If some softness is preferable, fold blankets carefully, making sure that they are even on each side and do not have awkward lumps and creases. Sometimes a large, fairly firm pillow or bolster is more convenient, although if one of these is too big, it can sometimes impede the success of the posture.
- Wear comfortable clothing that will not impede easy movement or make you feel constricted. A T-shirt and sweat pants or shorts is a popular combination. However, some people prefer leotards and tights. Avoid any garment with a tight waist. You should always practice yoga barefoot.

Practicing With Care

It is important to enjoy your yoga, and to maintain the balance and equilibrium that the discipline seeks to instill. Therefore, approach your practice with commitment, but also listen to your body.

- Even a few minutes of practice a day, or attending a class once a week, can bring positive change. But getting maximum benefit from yoga requires self-discipline and commitment.
- Do not, however, become so enthusiastic that your practice is self-destructive; understanding what you are doing is more important than achieving the next challenging position.
- Do not let effort and alertness turn into strain and tension. Learn to distinguish between normal discomfort, as your muscles stretch into new positions, and pain that may be warning you of imminent tissue damage.
- Respond intelligently to your own state when planning your practice. For example, if you have mild back or knee problems, you may be able to do most of the postures using support, or by not going into the full version of the pose.

Right Be realistic about what you hope to achieve with your yoga practice and don't feel you have to push yourself too hard.

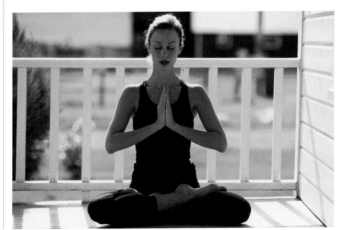

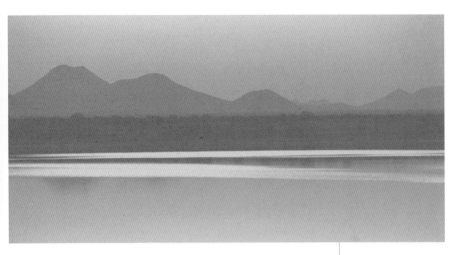

- If your injury is more serious, seek advice from an experienced yoga teacher, and check with your doctor if you are in any doubt about what you can do.
- Do not practice strenuously during menstruation. Avoid upside-down poses at that time, along with any that tighten, twist, or stretch the abdomen significantly.
- Practice on an empty stomach—wait about two hours after a full meal, one and a half after a snack.
- The morning can be a good time—after you have gone to the bathroom and before breakfast. Although the body is often stiffer when you have just got up, it is fresh, and your mind may be clearer than at the end of the day.
- Practicing when you feel mentally tired can also be very worthwhile and can restore energy.
- Use this book as a reference, reminder, and inspiration, but not as a lasting substitute for the watchful eye and responsive voice of a teacher. Working from a book, with a friend to check your position, can help you to avoid simple mistakes; however, more detailed instruction and individual adjustment can only come from the personal attention of someone who has studied yoga for many years. Guidance from an experienced teacher is particularly important if you have a medical condition, or experience pain or difficulty in the postures.

Above You will enjoy your yoga practice more if you are able to exercise in a tranquil, restful place. The quiet of the morning is a good time to practice.

23

Supporting Your Practice

Each posture has its own features, but in all of them, the parts of your body that are in contact with the floor are your foundation: the base on which the posture is built.

Opposite A wall might not seem to be the most obvious form of support in yoga, but it is remarkable how often one can help you with some of the supine or upside-down postures.

This base should be steady—so make sure you will not slip or wobble. Suggestions for using pieces of supporting equipment are included with the instructions for most postures in this book. If in doubt, use them—it is better to do the posture well and safely than stretch yourself too far and risk doing it incorrectly or injuriously.

Whenever you perform a posture, it is vital that you feel physically balanced and secure as you approach the completion of the movement. This means having good contact with the floor—or at least your mat—but also being able to "trust" the wall, chair, bolster, or whichever other item of support you select prior to doing the pose.

Caution
Seek medical advice before starting yoga, if you have any of the following conditions:
• Arthritis
• Cancer
• Detached retina
• Diabetes
• Epilepsy
• Heart condition
• High or low blood pressure
• Immune system disorder
• Ménière's disease
• Multiple sclerosis
• Myalgic encephalomyelitis
• Pregnancy or post-natal recovery
• Recent operation or accident

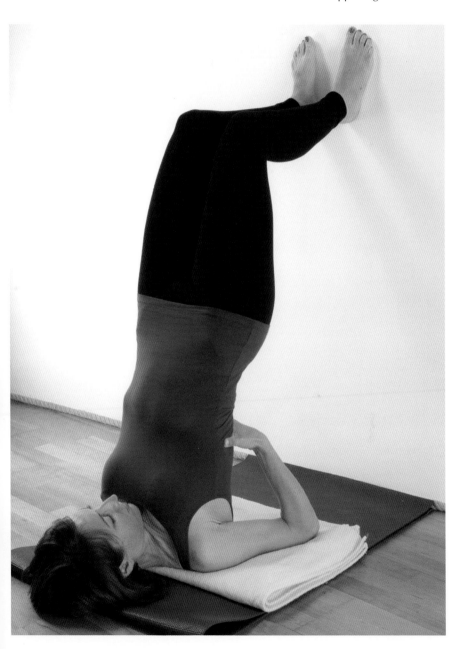

Developing a Program

Today, many people follow different exercise programs for varying reasons. Many contain elements of "truth" and are adpated to personal requirements. Yoga is about finding your own "truth" and can be a useful tool in your personal journey.

Opposite You might decide to make yoga your only form of exercise and then again, you might not. However you decide to approach the discipline, do so in a balanced and calm manner and seek inner mental peace as well as physical comfort and satisfaction.

The poet Kahlil Gibran encapsulated the proper outlook for yoga when he wrote:

"Say not, 'I have found the truth,' but rather, 'I have found a truth.' Say not, 'I have found the path of the soul.' Say rather, 'I have met the soul walking upon my path. For the soul walks upon all paths.'"

In this book, suggestions for building up a regular program of yoga practice are offered at the end, in the chapter entitled "Daily Routines," on pages 204–21. But these are suggestions only, designed to stimulate study and personal decisions. Some postures featured in this book do not appear in the "Daily Routines" chapter. However, this does not mean that they should not form a part of regular practice, but rather how they may fit in is a matter for personal decision. To build a program for yourself, take the following factors into consideration:

• So far as the physical aspect of postures is concerned, relate to your own body and its needs but do not necessarily regard a disinclination to practice something you find difficult as a message from the body. It might just be your mind feeling a little lazy!

• Bear in mind the principle of balance, which is at the core of yoga. The need for mental balance can affect which postures you choose to perform. The need for physical balance should determine the order in which they are performed. Many postures are always followed by a counter-posture. For instance, a stretch forward should be followed by a stretch backward.

- As you develop a daily program, constantly refer back—right to the beginning. You cannot remind yourself too often of the principles of yoga, and the different aspects of practice.

Starting Off

If you can, set aside a specific time each day for practice. Allow at least one and a half hours to digest a small snack or two hours for a meal before you begin. This applies to all postures, including breathing, visualization, and meditation. It is important to allow digestion to proceed unhampered.

- The length of your practice will depend on the time you have available and the postures you choose to include in your session. However, it is better to do ten minutes than to skip practice altogether.

- It makes sense to practice each new posture until you can remember the steps without needing to refer constantly to the instructions. It is wise to re-read the instructions from time to time to ensure that you are doing the posture correctly and have not left out steps.

- Some people may feel comfortable doing the same sequence each day, whereas others will prefer variety. In any case, right from the start, develop the habit of looking through the portion of the book you have studied, remind yourself of the points made, and then make your own choice of what you plan to do.

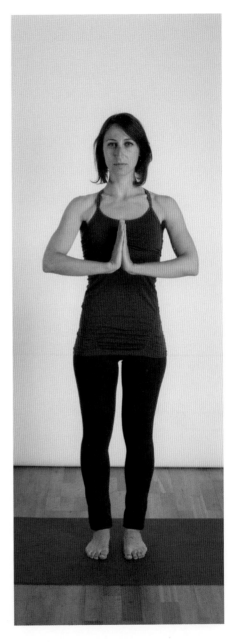

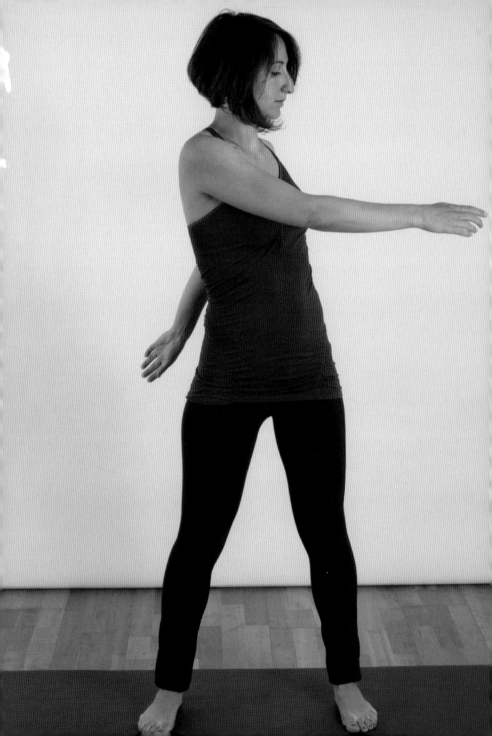

Getting Started

Yoga has something for everyone, regardless of your age and level of fitness. By reading this book and taking up this wonderful pastime, you are joining millions of people who enjoy and feel the myriad benefits of yoga in their everyday lives. Let's get started!

Breathing for Yoga

Breathing correctly and in a controlled manner is an integral part of yoga practice. Breath not only activates the body, it is also the basis of the functioning of the brain and mind. Although it is an automatic function, controlling the breath can enhance daily life.

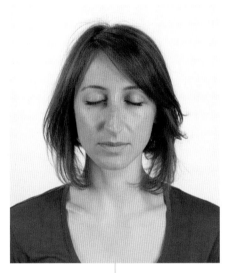

Above Practice your breathing regularly as well as the many postures featured in this book. Do not attempt Pranayama until you have some significant experience.

Worry, anger, agitation, and excitement all affect the way you breathe, interfering with the harmony and the flow of energy. Paying sensible attention to the way you breathe is the foundation of effective living.

The Breath of Life

Breath is life, but we also have great voluntary control over our breathing. The key to our energy system is in the diaphragm: a strong sheet of muscle, attached to the bottom ribs, separating the chest from the abdomen. The diaphragm acts as a piston, literally pumping the body's energy.

Breath Control

The yogic art of breath control is called Pranayama. Prana means "breath" but also denotes wind, the cosmic life force, energy, vitality, and the spirit or soul. Ayama means "extension," "regulation," "restraint," or "control." Thus, Pranayama signifies the prolongation and holding of the breath but also the direction and control of the vital energy that pervades every action, thought, and feeling. It is a powerful tool. In the ancient texts of yoga, regulating the breath has been likened to controlling a dangerous wild animal. The postures of yoga strengthen and prepare body and mind for breathing practices. Practice them for several months before you attempt Pranayama.

When and How to Practice Breathing

• Find a place where you will not be disturbed—somewhere clean, well-ventilated, and quiet.

• Practice breathing techniques in the morning (after using the bathroom and washing) and always on an empty stomach.

• Do not try the techniques immediately after exercise (including yoga), that have an exhausting or disturbing effect.

• If you are depressed or distressed, do not practice breathing exercises, but choose postures that you know from experience will lighten your mood.

• If you feel strained or start to panic during controlled breathing, return to breathing normally and rest.

• Lie down to practice, with support under the back (see page 128). At first, a few minutes will be enough. After breath control practice, rest lying flat in the Corpse pose (see pages 129–31), and do not do other postures.

For much more information on breathing for yoga, see pages 134–39.

Caution
• Do not underestimate the often very powerful effects of breathing and meditative practices. Seek the guidance of a yoga teacher before embarking on regular or sustained practice.
• Certain breathing techniques should not be practiced at all during pregnancy, so if you are pregnant, make sure your teacher knows. Any techniques that involve holding the breath need special care.
• Stop if you feel tightness or heaviness in the chest, your breathing sounds harsh, or speeds up, you are getting short of breath, your head is becoming hot.

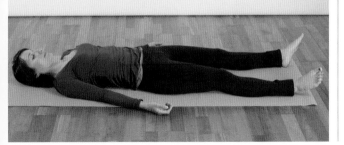

Left Relaxing in the Corpse pose (see pages 129–31) is one great way to practice your breathing.

31

General Stretching

The first areas of the body to stiffen up are the back, neck, and shoulders. This is because the muscles in these areas of the body respond quickly to tension and poor posture.

T he good news is that a range of simple, general stretching movements will ease these areas if they are performed little and often. The exercises should ideally become a regular part of your yoga practice.

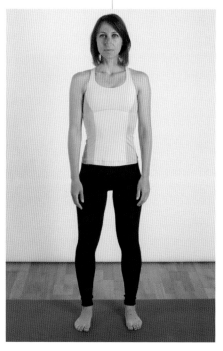

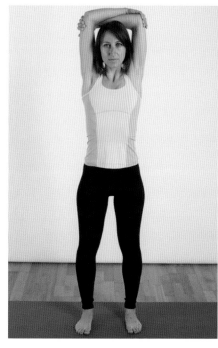

1 Stand tall in Mountain pose.

2 As you inhale, raise both hands above the head; lift through the fingertips as though you are trying to touch something just out of reach. Take hold of your elbows.

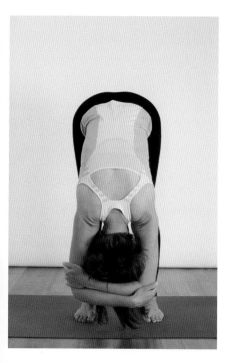 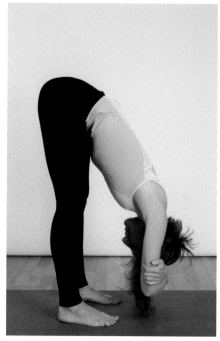

3 On an exhale, allow the arms to swing forward and carry you into a Forward Fold. Keep your arms folded over each other on the top of your head. Keep the knees slightly bent so as not to strain your back.

4 Inhale, lift back up to standing and separate the feet a little wider than hip distance apart; both feet stay facing forward. Allow the arms to swing freely as you swing from side to side.

Warming Up

Never forget that stretching and general warming up of the body is a form of exercise in its own right, which can be conducted either as languidly or as vigorously as you see fit. However you choose to stretch, and however often you do it, ensure that you begin gently and let your muscles and joints literally warm to the task. You will find all yoga postures easier and more comfortable to perform if you take the trouble to stretch and warm up properly at the outset.

Relaxing the Spine

In the human anatomy, the spine is tremendously important. It provides essential flexibility and support, and it also provides a vital channel for the nerves, while its alignment affects the functioning of important muscles. We allow it to stiffen, or become distorted, at our peril. When performing yoga movements for the spine, always remember that the body functions as a whole.

The Cat

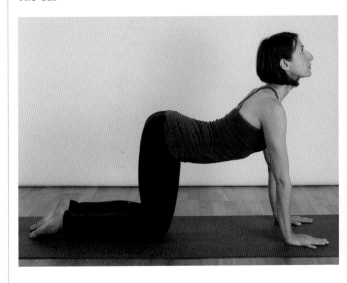

1 Drop on to all fours, knees a little apart, palms facing forward beneath the shoulder blades. Breathe in, dropping the back, and raising the head. Hold for several seconds.

Considering the Whole Body

When exercising an individual part of the body, you must still consider the whole. Working on the spine is working on the entire being. Some stretches are slow dynamic movements; the Spinal Twist is a static one. Each has its own special benefits.

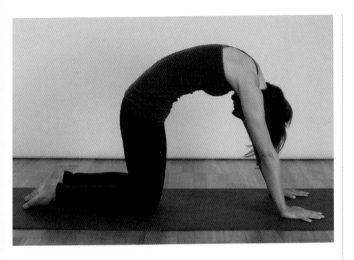

2 Breathing out, arch the back as high as it will go, dropping the head between the arms. Again, hold the position for a number of seconds. Repeat between 10 and 20 times.

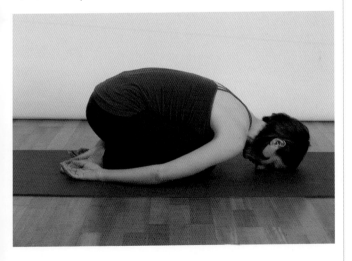

3 Finally, sink back on the heels, hands by the feet, palms facing upward, forehead touching the ground. Remain relaxed for two or three minutes. Get up quietly and slowly.

35

The Back Body Stretch

"Back" here refers to the whole posterior part of the body. You have to remember that you are constantly subject to the force of gravity. Over the years this can compress the body and needs to be countered by effective stretching. The Back Body Stretch works from the fingers to the toes: stretching the back of the body and compressing the front of the trunk. The majority of people allow the back to become stiff. The more the mind dwells on stiffness, the greater the problem becomes. Do not regard the pose either as difficult or easy; just say to yourself, "I am doing it"—and follow the instructions carefully.

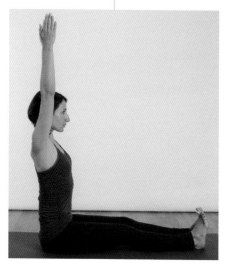

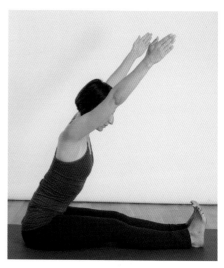

1 Sit on the floor with the legs out in front, feet a few inches apart, toes pointing upward. Let the hands rest on the floor, palms down by the sides. Breathe slowly out and then, as you inhale, stretch the arms right up in the air, lifting the trunk. This will stretch the spine and the back muscles.

2 As you breathe out, stretch slowly forward, maintaining the extended back, keeping the arms straight and the back of the legs on the floor. Breath and movement should come together exactly and the only thought should be one of reaching forward.

36

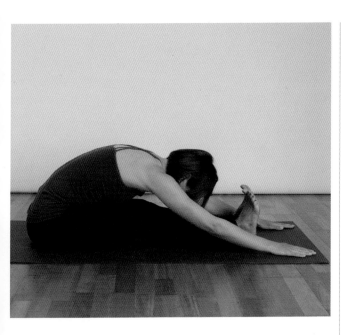

Helpful Hint
Think about the torso slowly moving forward, as opposed to downward, and the lower abdomen moving toward the upper thighs, rather than dropping the head to the knees.

3 As the out-breath ends, let the hands hold the farthest part they can reach: the toes, the feet, the ankles, or even the calves. Maintain a relaxed stretch with head hanging down. Hold, breathing gently, for at least 30 seconds. Come back up, breathing in.

Removing Stiffness
This is a position which many people find difficult, but if you concentrate on the difficulty you will never progress. In most cases lower-back stiffness comes from lack of use and the muscles are perfectly capable of stretching. The same applies to the hamstrings. Right from the start, perform this asana quietly and slowly, and do not let considerations of time affect you. If you do experience any back problems while performing this posture, take a break from it for a while and, if you are at all concerned, consult both your doctor and your yoga instructor. The latter may be able to find alternative poses for you.

37

Easy Sun Salutation

Since ancient times, the sun has always been a source of both worship and reverence. In this practice, we give thanks to the power and vitality of the sun. The flow of movement takes the body in all directions, working on all the major joint and muscle groups as well as toning the abdominal organs. Start by holding each position for a breath or two, reduce to one full breath in each pose.

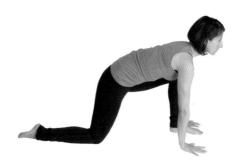

6 Hands to floor

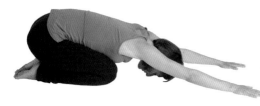

5 Child's pose

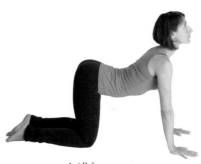

4 All fours, cat pose

Aim for 5–10 complete rounds. If this is all you have time for, a sun salutation, followed by a short time in Savasana (Corpse pose) is a great practice on its own. When you have completed these first six positions, repeat the sequence on the other side with the following very slight variation in the order of postures: 7 Kneel, hands in prayer; 8 Left foot forward to lunge; 9 Hands to floor; 10 All fours, cow pose. 11 Child's pose; 12 Return to kneel.

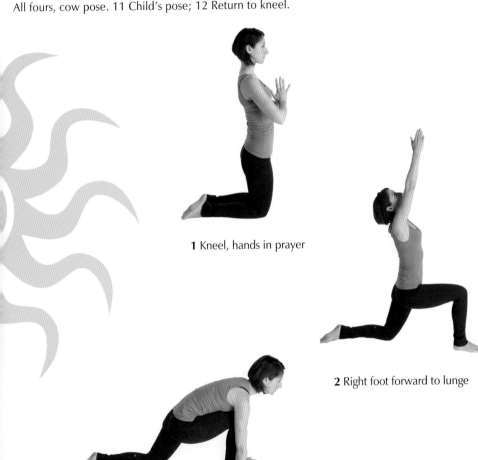

1 Kneel, hands in prayer

2 Right foot forward to lunge

3 Bow hands to floor

39

Advanced Sun Salutation

As before, follow the sequence below and repeat as many times as you are able to or have time for. Rest in the Corpse pose when you feel you have had enough of these successive postures.

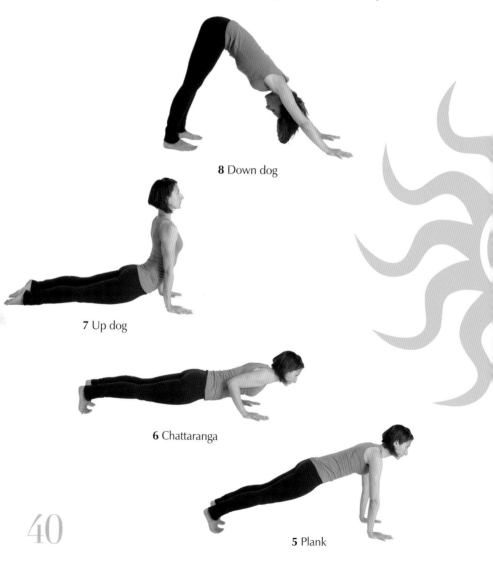

8 Down dog

7 Up dog

6 Chattaranga

5 Plank

When you have completed these first eight positions, repeat the sequence with the following very slight variation: 9 Plank; 10 Chattaranga; 11 Uttanasana; 12 Raise hands to sky.

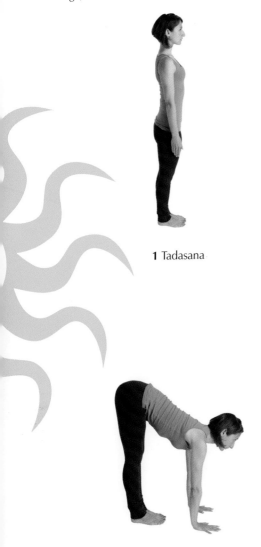

1 Tadasana

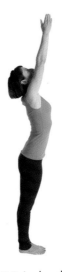

2 Raise hands

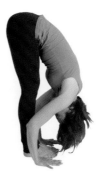

3 Uttanasana

4 Raise chest

41

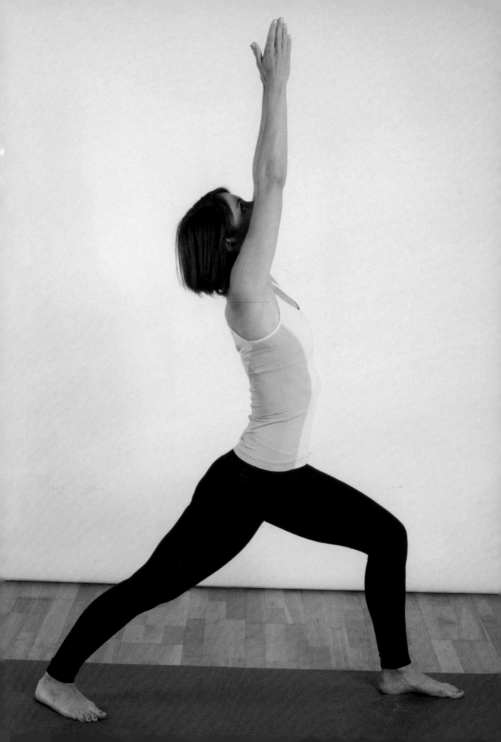

Standing Postures

Regular practice of standing postures can change the way you feel and how you appear to others. They are active, stimulating poses that warm the muscles, promote healthy breathing and circulation, and lift your mood. These elegant postures help to develop strength, poise, and coordination. They stretch the legs; bring mobility to hips, shoulders, and spine; and increase stability and confidence. These poses improve spatial awareness—important for more complex yoga postures and a protection against injury.

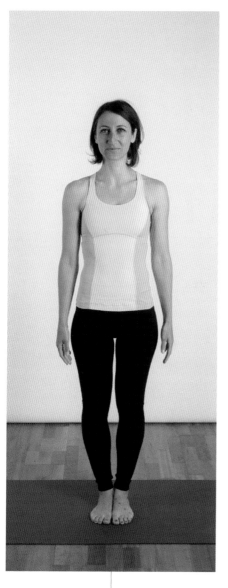

Tadasana — The Mountain

Tadasana creates the strong foundations through the feet that we require for all of the standing yoga poses.

1 Stand with your feet together if you can, or ever so slightly apart if this is more comfortable. Close your eyes and rock very gently from side to side rolling on the soles of the feet, then rock backward and forward from heels to toes. Come to rest at the place that feels the most balanced. Open your eyes.

2 With straight legs, engage your thigh muscles above the knee, so that it feels as if the thighs are lifting up. The knee should have a micro bend, so that the knee joint itself is soft and the knee is not over extended. Take the top of the thigh bones gently back in space so your weight is stacked over the ankles.

3 Lengthen the sides of the waist and continue

to feel the lift up through the ribcage and heart, create space in the upper chest, taking the shoulders back, and the shoulder blades down the back. Keep the stomach muscles engaged, as if you are pulling the abdomen into the lower back while the shoulders and arms remain relaxed. The arms hang naturally.

4 Gently lengthen the neck as if you are lifting through the crown of the head and balance the back of the head in line with the heels. Look forward and try to keep the face relaxed. Soften your lips.

Lifting the Chest

When we feel depressed, we have a tendency to hunch our shoulders or "droop." When we feel happy, the chest lifts and we stand tall. By consciously lifting the chest we can create a sense of openness in the body that instantly lifts the mood. When the chest rises and the ribcage is open, we can breathe deeper, which makes the mind feel clearer and improves our frame of mind.

Helpful Hint
To give the pose extra power, raise your arms above your head and touch palms. Keep your neck long and your shoulders down. Reach as high as you can and enjoy the stretch.

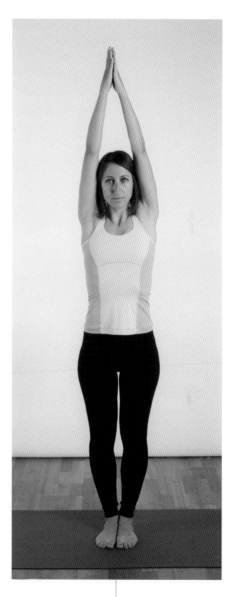

Utkatasana — The Chair

This posture has an obvious strengthening effect on the legs and the back. Its name, Utkatasana, means "powerful" or "fierce." It is like lifting up from sitting on a chair—an image you may find helpful when performing it. It develops strong legs, builds stamina, and strengthens willpower and determination.

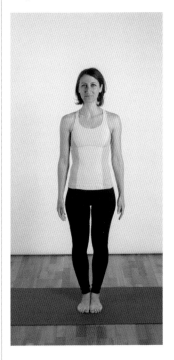 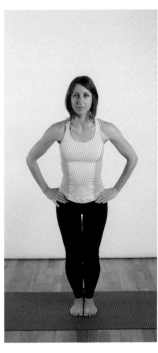

1 Stand tall in Tadasana (see pages 44–5) with the gaze forward.

2 Deeply bend both knees as if you are going to sit down on a chair; you can bring the hands onto the waist to stabilize yourself if you need to. Rock your weight back to the heels of the feet, but keep the toes on the floor.

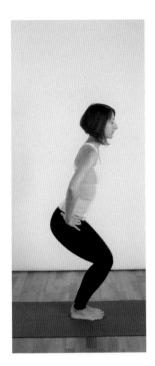
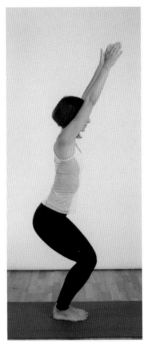
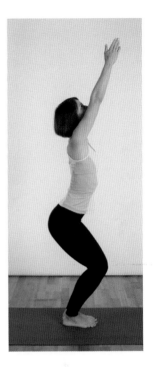

3 Lift up out of the hips with the torso, so that the sides of the waist are long and the chest is lifted.

4 Extend the arms alongside the ears and gaze up toward your fingertips, but keep the back of the neck long. Press palms together, or for tight shoulders, have the palms facing in about shoulder distance apart. See if you can lower the shoulder blades away from the ears.

5 Hold the pose and gaze up toward your fingertips while breathing deeply.

Helpful Hint
Remember that the upper body stays light and lifts away from the thighs.

47

Vrksasana — The Tree

As we physically balance the body, so we bring balance to the mind. In this pose, if our thoughts are all over the place, our tree will be as well! Consequently, we have to focus on our balance, and that immediately brings clarity and a sense of calm.

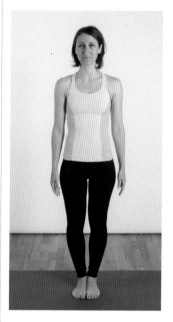 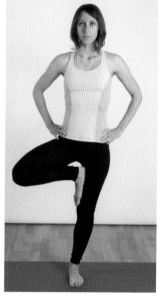

1 Stand in Tadasana (see pages 44–5) with the feet together or slightly apart. As you exhale, begin to shift your weight over on to the left leg, holding a steady gaze out in front of you.

2 As you inhale, start to lift the right leg up off the floor, reach down with your right hand, and take hold of the ankle. Guide it to the top of the left thigh and press the sole of the foot against the leg to hold it in place.

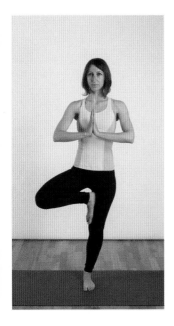
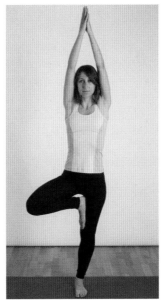

3 Bring both hands together or to the waist to help you balance. Soften the knee of the standing leg and engage the thigh muscles so that the knee is protected. Engage your stomach muscles to create strength and stability in the pose.

4 On an inhale, raise both arms straight up, with the palms facing. Either bring the palms to touch, or for tight shoulders, keep the hands wider apart. Lift from the abdomen, the sides of the waist and the ribcage rather than from the shoulders.

Variations
- This pose is easier to perform if you do not lift the arms; the hands can stay on the waist or you can press palms into a prayer position.
- If the foot will not come to the top of the thigh, bring it to the middle of your calf, or keep the toes on the ground and lift the heel to just above the ankle on the standing leg.
- Hold for 8–10 slow, deep breaths, and release by taking the left hand back down to the ankle and then gently down to the floor.

49

Garudasana—The Eagle

This pose is named after Garuda, the giant man-eagle of Indian mythology, who transported the god Vishnu. In this pose, the entwining of the legs and the arms stretches the back of the hips and the upper back more than most other elementary postures. It is good for opening the shoulders and easing stiffness in them, while benefiting the hips and legs as well.

1 Stand in Tadasana (see pages 44–5).

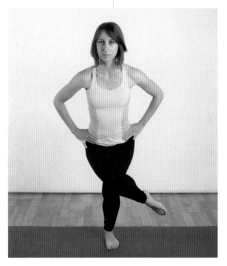 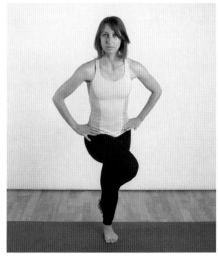

2 Bend both knees and shift your weight on to your left leg. Lift the right leg over the left and cross the legs above the knee. The right toes hook around the back of the left calf and rest on the inner shin. Relax the toes of the standing leg.

3 If this position creates pain in the knee, release the toes and just stay with the cross above the knee. Squeeze your inner thighs together. Cross the legs above the knee.

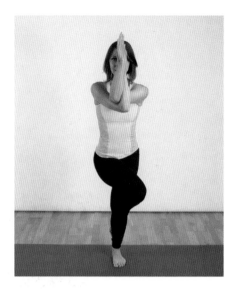 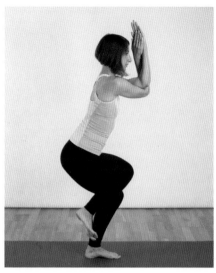

4 Hook the right toes around the back of your left calf. Take the arms out at shoulder height and cross the left arm over the right above the elbow. Take the fingertips of both up toward the ceiling. With little fingers away from the face, bring the right fingertips to touch the left palm.

5 Lower the shoulder blades down away from the ears and lift the elbows so that they line up with the tops of the shoulders. Soften your gaze and look past your hands.

Variation
As a variation to the pose, sit down lower to make it more challenging. Fold forward.

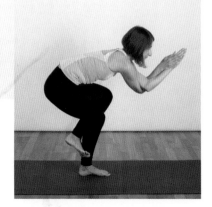

Trikonasana – The Triangle

The name of this posture reveals its shape. It is a fundamental standing pose that strengthens spine and abdominal muscles.

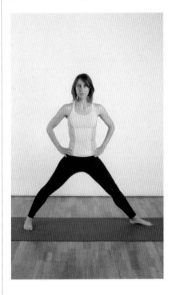 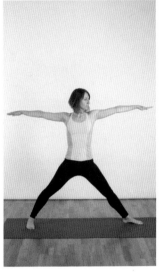

1 Stand in Tadasana (see pages 44–5). Step back with your right foot so that the heels are in line (you can use the edge of your mat to judge this). There should be roughly the distance of one of your leg lengths between the heels. The left toes stay facing the front of the mat, the right toes are diagonal to the mat, at about a 45° angle. Square your hips and shoulders forward as pictured.

2 Use your stomach muscles to press down through the soles of the feet and lift a little higher through the crown of the head. Keep the toes relaxed. Both legs are straight. Lift the thigh muscles up toward the pelvis. Extend both arms out to shoulder height.

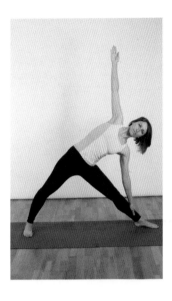 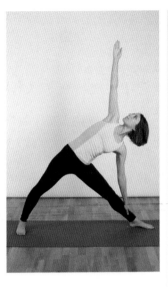

Helpful Hint
Try to roll your left hip under and your outer right thigh back. Use your stomach muscles to press back to the outside edge of the back foot.

3 Take your left arm gently forward so that you start to feel the beginning of a stretch on the inner left thigh, then drop the left hand down toward the shin bone and rest it there. Over time, try to take the weight out of the left hand, so that you are using your stomach muscles to support the pose and not your left arm or hand.

4 Turn your right palm to face toward the top of your head and turn the gaze up toward the palm of the hand. If this causes strain or discomfort for the neck, look down toward the left toes. Hold for 25–45 seconds or for 5–8 slow, deep breaths. Repeat on the other side.

Using Support
Use a block for the left hand if necessary, to keep the weight even on both feet.

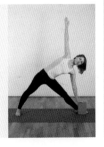

53

Parsvakonasana—The Horizon

This posture causes you to stretch sideways, but its Sanskrit name Parsvakonasana can also refer to the line where earth and sky meet, so the posture is a reminder that yoga extends your horizons.

1 Stand in Tadasana (see pages 44–5).

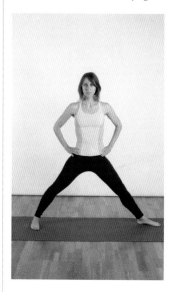 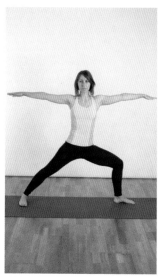

2 Inhale. Come into triangle pose (see pages 52–3), bring your hands to your waist and square the hips forward.

3 Exhale. Bend your left knee over your heel, keeping the left toes relaxed. Inhale, and extend your arms up to shoulder height.

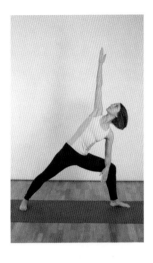 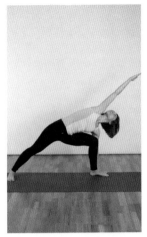 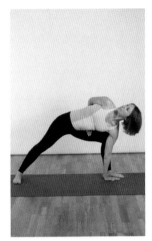

4 Exhale. Bring the left elbow to rest on the left knee, raise the right arm straight up into the air, and look up to the palm of your right hand. If you are comfortable here, take the left hand to a block or all the way down to the floor on the outside edge of the left foot. The forearm and the shin bone should be in line.

5 Optionally, take the right arm alongside the right ear, stretch from the sides of the waist and not just from the shoulder. The stretch should run from the back right heel all the way to the fingertips. If the neck is OK to do so, look to your fingertips on your right hand; alternatively, gaze straight ahead or downward.

6 Press the outer shin against the inner arm to spiral the chest open to the ceiling or sky. Engage the stomach muscles and press back to the outside edge of the back heel, keeping the weight even on both feet and re-establishing stability into the pose.

Variation
Hand inside foot, take right arm behind back, hook to upper left thigh for a deeper twist.

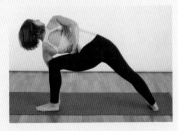

Virabhadrasana I – The Warrior I

Your arms are your swords: they should be as strong as steel and unwavering as they extend out from the shoulders.

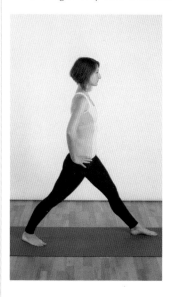 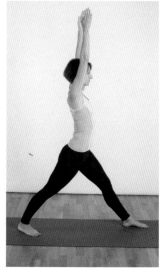

1 Stand in Mountain pose (see pages 44–5). Inhale, bring your hands to the waist, and step the right foot straight back, keeping the heels in line. Left foot points forward, right foot turns out 45°.

2 Move the right hip forward while pushing the left hip back if necessary to square the hips to the front of the mat. Inhale to raise both arms straight up alongside the ears. Drop the shoulders down, away from the ears. Press your weight to the outside edge of the back heel.

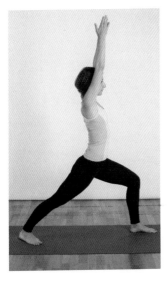 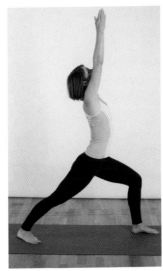

3 Exhale and bend your left knee to a right angle. The left shin and trunk should remain vertical. Press into the floor with your left heel.

4 Sink down a little so that the left knee bends deeper. Hold for 10–12 long, deep breaths. To come out of the pose, bring the hands back to the waist, deeply bend the left knee, and step forward.

Helpful Hints

- Keeping your hands on the hips is less strenuous. It can also help if your lower back hurts when your arms are raised—but seek guidance from a yoga teacher if you suffer back pain.
- Discomfort in the lumbar region can sometimes be eased by making sure your hips are level and well turned to the side and by stretching up so that your waist does not shorten.
- If you find it impossible to turn the back foot in and keep the heel down, place a small support—such as a wooden wedge or folded blanket—under the heel.

Virabhadrasana II—The Warrior II

The second Warrior pose, Virabhadrasana II, is a vigorous posture that strengthens the legs and back. These challenging positions help to develop fortitude and stamina. Don't approach them with brutality and gritted teeth, however, but with persistence, sensitivity, and care —the qualities of a truly noble warrior.

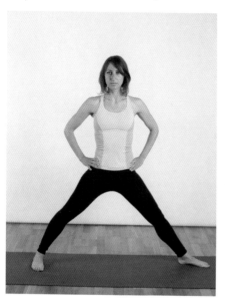 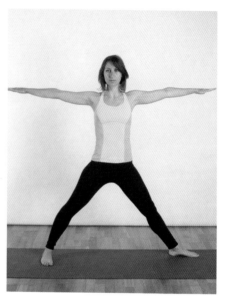

1 Stand in Mountain pose (see pages 44–5). Inhale, bring your hands to waist, and step back into Triangle pose (see pages 52–3). Square your hips and shoulders forward.

2 Raise your arms to shoulder height. Do not disturb the position of your upper body nor the balance of your arms as you turn your feet.

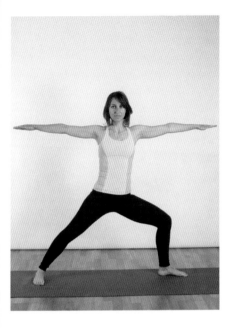
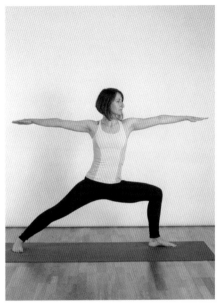

3 Exhaling, lower your hips, and bend your left knee to a right angle. The left shin and the trunk should be vertical, the inner left thigh stretching toward the knee. The right leg stays firm and straight, the knee facing forward and the outer edge of the right heel pressing down. The trunk faces forward, stretching upward evenly. To prevent leaning sideways, concentrate on lifting both the right and left sides of your waist. Do not lean forward or backward, but lift the front chest and the back ribs. Stretch your arms to the right and to the left, parallel to the floor and in line with each other.

4 Keeping awareness in the stretch of your arms, turn your head and look to the left. Make sure you do not bring your neck out of line, nor hunch your shoulders. This is an expansive pose. Face and throat should be relaxed, with comfortable breathing. Stay in the posture for 20–30 seconds. Inhaling, come up and face forward. You may need to rest your arms before repeating on the other side. Finally, jump your feet together and lower the arms.

Namaste — The Prayer

Joining the palms of the hands is a gesture of prayer in many cultures. In India, this gesture, known as Namaste, is a sign of respect, used in greeting, paying homage, and acknowledging a gift. The right and left hands can be said to represent our active and passive sides, so joining them evenly can suggest the harmonization of these complementary opposites in our nature. Normally the Namaste takes place in front of the body, but here it is done at the back. The Prayer position brings mobility to the shoulders and arms, encouraging the chest to open and the breathing to improve.

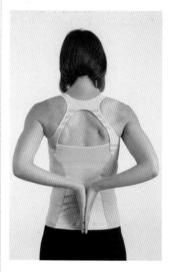 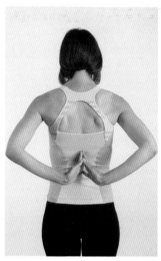

1 Join your palms behind the center of your back, fingers pointing down.

2 Turn your fingers in toward your spine and then up, keeping your shoulders and elbows back.

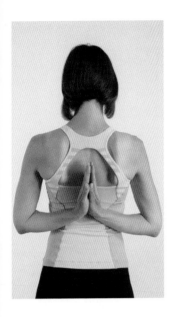
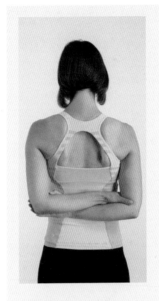

3 Take your hands higher up your back so that your wrists are higher than your elbows. The outer upper arms stretch down; the forearms stretch up. Extend all your fingers so they contact their counterparts along their whole length, and press together the base of each palm.

Alternative

If the full pose is too difficult, you can still encourage openness in the chest by clasping your elbows behind you and drawing the shoulders back.

61

Prasarita Padottanasana—Forward Bend, Feet Wide

In this pose, the feet are widely spread and the legs strongly stretched. When the full posture is assumed, with the head on the floor, it has some of the benefits of a headstand—without the challenge of balancing! Its Sanskrit name, derives from the words for "expanded," "foot," or "leg" and "extended."

1 Stand in Tadasana (see pages 44–5).

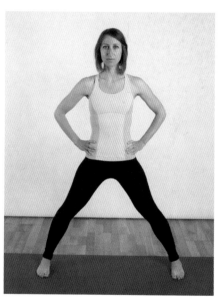

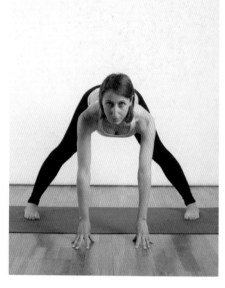

2 Step your feet wide and bring your hands to hips. Check that your feet are level and parallel, facing forward. Do not tip onto either the outer or inner edges of your feet, but lift both sides of your ankles. Keep your spine lifting, legs straight, and your front thigh muscles firmly pulled up.

3 Exhale and bend forward from your hips to take your hands to the floor, placing them shoulder-width apart. With arms straight, extend the front of your body, and make your back concave. Look up without straining your neck or hunching your shoulders.

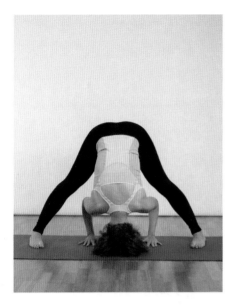

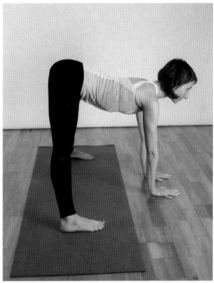

4 Keeping your legs straight and vertical, take your trunk farther down and place the top of your head on the floor. To do this, move your hands back in line with your feet, and bend your elbows, keeping your arms parallel. Lift your hips and relax your trunk.

5 Stay for about 30 seconds, then inhale, and raise your trunk to the concave position, straightening your arms. Place your hands on your hips, stand up, and bring your feet together.

Using Support
- If your head cannot reach the floor, try resting it on foam blocks.
- If your hands cannot reach the floor without causing your back to round or your knees to bend, place your hands on blocks or on a chair.

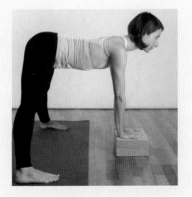

63

Adho Mukha Savanasana—The Dog

Animals know how to release muscle tension naturally, and this posture recalls how dogs and cats sometimes stretch. It relieves stiffness in the lower legs, making it especially valuable if you spend a lot of time standing, walking, or running. It also restores energy and rests the heart while still having an invigorating effect. It is grouped with the standing poses because it has much in common with them.

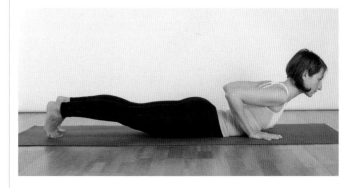

1 Lie on the floor, face down, with your feet about hip-width apart, toes tucked under. Place your hands on each side of your chest, fingers slightly spread and pointing forward.

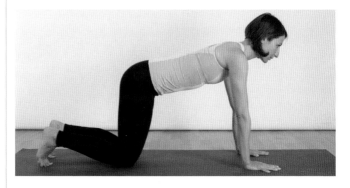

2 Come up onto your hands and knees, straightening your arms. Check that your hands are level and all the fingers are pressing down.

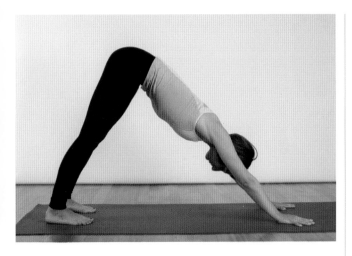

Variation

This posture uses many parts of the body and can relieve stiff necks and shoulders. Although it often makes other postures easier, the Dog pose is a challenging stretch at first. If your heels cannot reach the ground, work with them pressing on a wall.

3 Lift your hips and straighten your legs completely, taking your heels down toward the floor. To do this, stretch the sole back from the ball of each foot evenly, keeping your feet parallel, and move shins and thighs back. The hands stay firmly pressing down. Stretch all your fingers and make sure the roots of your index finger and thumb are well grounded.

4 Make sure your arms are straight; all four limbs should be strong so that you can stretch your trunk up. Draw your shoulder blades down the back, opening your chest and armpits. Relax your head and neck, breathe evenly, and stay for 30–60 seconds before coming down from the pose.

Using Support
For additional support, place your thumbs and index fingers against the wall, and rest your head on a pad, such as a folded blanket or foam block. Supporting the head increases the rejuvenating effect of the pose, provided you do not sink your body weight heavily into your head.

65

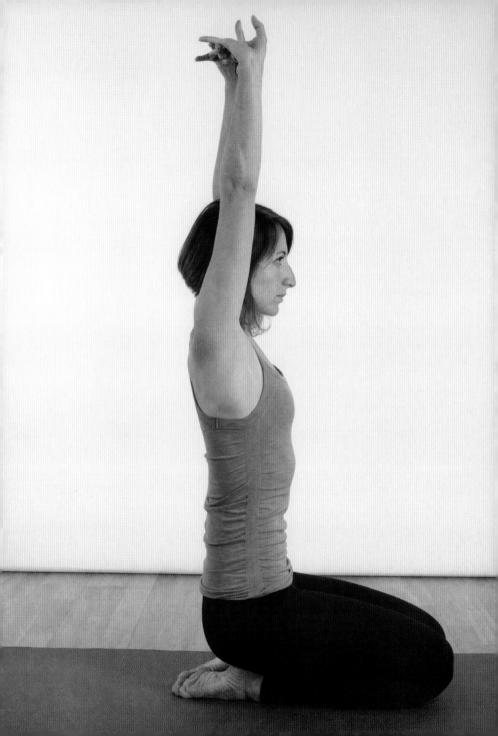

Sitting Postures

Sitting poses continue the work of strengthening and stretching the body, but in a less vigorous way—although the effects can be just as intense. Most of the postures are calming, but they still need concentration and precision. A few more demanding positions can call for perseverance—and maybe some help from supports. Several of the poses encourage flexibility in the legs, hips, and back and may need to be modified if you are stiff or have suffered an injury and feel strain in the knees or back. Never persist with any posture that is painful.

Dandasana—The Staff

The staff or rod is a symbol of support, strength, uprightness, and authority. In this pose, called Dandasana in Sanskrit, the staff is the spine itself—upright and supportive. This simple posture is the basis of the sitting poses, strengthening the back and teaching you how to work the legs, even though you are not standing on them.

- Sit on the floor, with your legs stretched out together in front. Place your hands on the floor behind you.
- Straighten your legs completely, joining your feet and keeping the center of the back of each leg facing the floor.
- Keep your feet upright—without tensing the tops of them—and the front thigh muscles firm.
- Your spine should be erect, shoulders back, and chest open. The lower back should lift and the waist should stay long.
- Stay for about 30 seconds in the pose, keeping neck, face, and breathing relaxed.

Using Support
- If there is tightness in the hamstrings or weakness in the back, it may be difficult to lift properly—the back may slump and the front of the trunk shorten. To avoid this, sit on a firm pad or folded blanket. The support raises the hips and makes the angle between trunk and legs less acute, so you can stretch up the spine more easily.
- Prepare yourself for forward bending by placing a belt around your feet and holding each end of it. Pull on the belt with straight arms, gripping at a distance from the feet that allows your back to be upright.

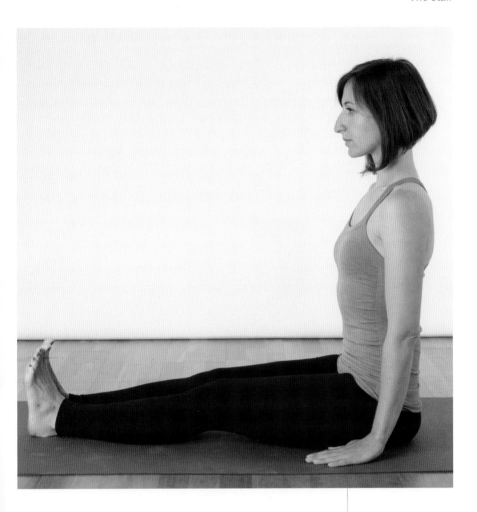

Paschimottansana—Seated Forward Bend

This pose is one of the most important postures of yoga. It provides an intense stretch in the back of the body, while at the same time quieting the mind. The backs of the legs are lengthened as well as the spine. Viewing the body as a microcosm, the head is at the north, the lower body is the south, the front is the east, and the back is the west. The back of the body is an area that we do not see and may be less aware of, like our unconscious self, which yoga also challenges.

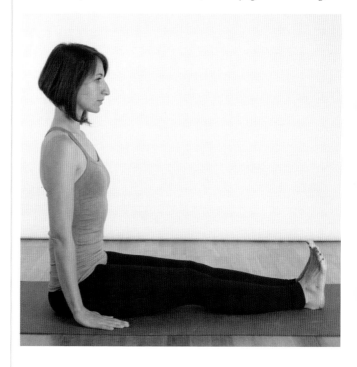

1 Sit in the Staff pose (see pages 68–9) stretching up your spine.

2 Exhale and lean forward to catch your feet, keeping the legs completely straight. Raise your head and lift your chest, with straight arms and a concave action on the back, so it stays flat. Here, the legs are stretching, and the spine is erect.

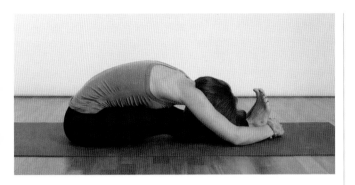

3 To go farther, on another exhalation take your trunk down onto your legs, head resting on your shins, and hands clasping beyond your feet if you can. Stretch the front, sides, and back of your trunk and keep the backs of your knees down. Stay in the pose for 30 seconds.

Using Support
- Sitting on folded blankets makes the posture easier, especially if your legs or lower back are stiff. Add height if your lower back still slumps backward. Let your waist lengthen, and the lower ribs move away from the pelvic rim.
- It is hard to reach the feet at first and more important that you keep the legs extended. Use a belt around your feet to hold on to.

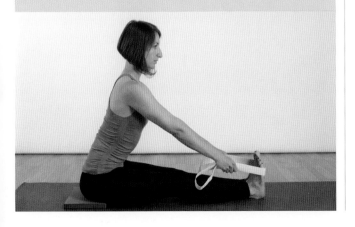

Virasana—The Hero

This is a posture of quiet alertness, suitable for breathing and meditative practices. It takes its Sanskrit name, Virasana, from Vira, meaning "a hero."

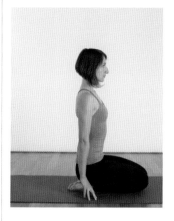
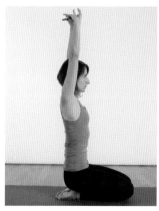

Helpful Hints
• If pressure on the top of your feet is painful, kneel on a blanket.

• If you cannot stretch the fronts of your ankles, place a rolled cloth underneath them.

• If you cannot lower your bottom to your heels, sit on a rolled or folded blanket.

Easy Version: Sitting On Heels
1 Kneel down so you can sit on your feet and keep your knees together. Place your feet evenly on the floor, with your heels separated, and your big toes closer together.

2 Sit upright, balanced equally over your right and left sides. Stretch up your trunk, shoulders back, hands by your sides on the floor to help you lift. Do not lean forward or backward, or let your spine slump. Stay for a minute or two in this posture.

With Arms Stretching Up: Parvatasana
You can make the posture more active and lift the trunk more by stretching up your arms.

1 Interlock your fingers, then turn your thumbs toward you and down, so your palms face away.

2 Straighten your arms fully and stretch them up, without poking your lower ribs forward. Hold for several seconds, then bring your hands down and interlock your fingers again but with the other index finger on top. Repeat the stretch up.

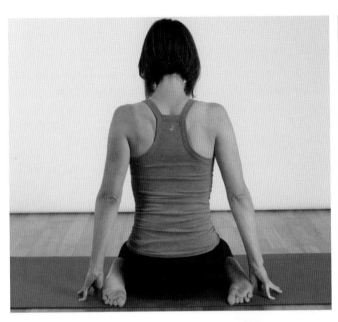

Caution
Do not ignore any pain in your knees; they are vulnerable joints.

Using Support
• Take a pad and place it between your feet.
• Kneel with your toes pointing straight back and the center fronts of your feet on the floor. Try to get all the toes in contact with the floor.
• Sit down on the pad between your feet and stretch the trunk up. In this and in the full pose, you can also stretch up your arms and bend forward.

Preparing for the Full Posture
Eventually, in the Hero pose, you sit on the floor between your feet. Because this can be a strain on the knees, do not attempt the full posture if you feel any pain. In the full posture, your bottom is firmly on the floor, but you may need to support your bottom above floor level at first.

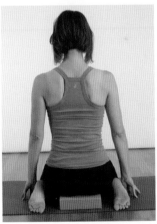

73

Gomukhasana — Cow's Head

The Cow's Head pose is effective at mobilizing the shoulder joints and stretching the top chest. In the full posture, you cross your legs underneath your trunk, but it is also beneficial to do the arm movements separately—either standing, sitting in the Hero (see pages 72–3) or Easy Cross-Legged position (see pages 78–9), or kneeling (as shown here).

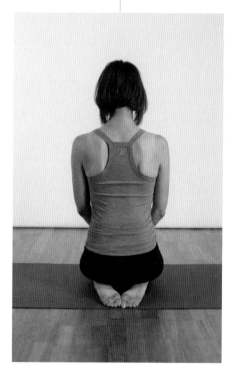

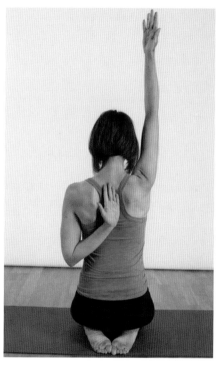

1 Sit comfortably in the easy version of the Hero pose, with your bottom resting on your heels. Breathe deeply and relax.

2 With an upright trunk, take your left arm behind your back, palm facing out, and bend your elbow so the fingers point up your spine. Move your hand high up between the shoulder blades, still with your palm out, keeping your shoulder back.

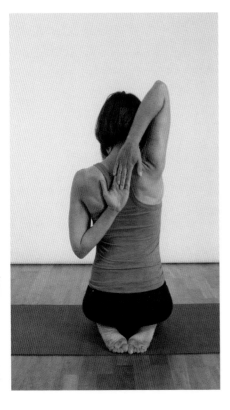

Helpful Hints
- If you cannot join hands, use a belt or scarf to make a connection between them.
- Once you have linked your fingers, continue to work over the months to hold farther along your hands.

3 Stretch your right arm up, bend your elbow, and bring your hand down to clasp your left hand. Your top elbow points straight up and your chest is evenly lifted.

4 Stay for 30 seconds or more, then release your hands, and repeat with the hand and arm positions reversed.

Balasana—Child's Pose

The Child's Pose move stretches your lower back and arms and relaxes your entire body. If you have knee problems, lower yourself into this yoga pose with extra care.

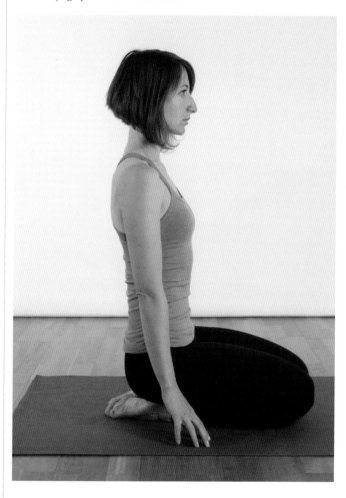

1 Sit comfortably in the easy version of the Hero pose, with your bottom resting on your heels. Breathe deeply and relax.

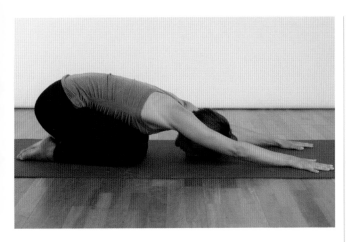

2 Lower your bottom toward your heels as you stretch the rest of your body down and forward. Extend the arms out in front of your head and bring your forehead to the mat.

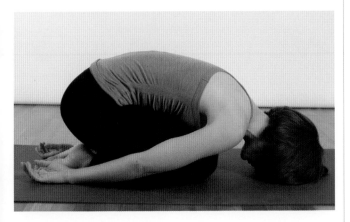

3 In the fully stretched position, rest your arms in a relaxed position along the floor, rest your stomach comfortably on top of your thighs, and rest your forehead on the mat.

4 You should feel a mild stretch in your shoulders and buttocks and down the length of your spine and arms.

Sukhasana — Easy Cross-Legged Pose

This position derives its Sanskrit name, Sukhasana, from the word sukha, meaning "easy" or "pleasant." It also refers to aspiring after future virtue. When you become discouraged by more difficult postures, it is agreeable to return to this one. It can be a reminder that, although the path is long and hard, there are resting places from which to gaze ahead with equanimity. This posture can be used for breathing exercises and meditation.

1 Sit in the Staff pose (see pages 68–9).

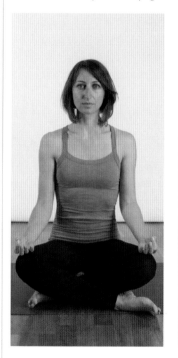 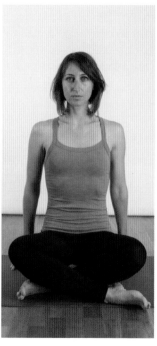

2 Bend your legs and cross your shins, so each foot is under the opposite leg and your knees are off the floor.

3 Press your hands into the floor on each side of you to lift your spine up.

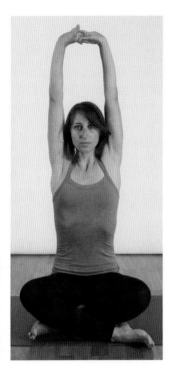

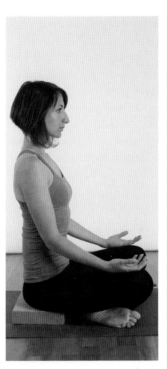

Helpful Hints
- It is difficult to keep your trunk lifting, especially if your hips are stiff, so sit on a foam block or a folded blanket to improve the posture.
- Stretching your arms up can also improve the stretch.

4 Have even weight on each buttock and keep your shoulders level and relaxed, chest open. You can rest your hands on your knees. Reach upward to improve the stretch.

5 Hold for about a minute, then cross your legs the other way, and repeat. Sitting on a foam block or a folded blanket will ease the completion of this posture.

Baddha Konasana—The Tailor

A position adopted by craftworkers in some parts of the world, this posture can help urinary and gynecological conditions and is also used for meditation. Its name, Baddha Konasana, describes the shape of the pose (baddha means "restrained" or "bound," kona means "angle"). It also recalls the philosophical view that we are bound by our human existence, our failings, and personal history. Beyond its usefulness as a system of exercise, yoga can be a means of understanding those restrictions—ultimately enabling us to transcend them.

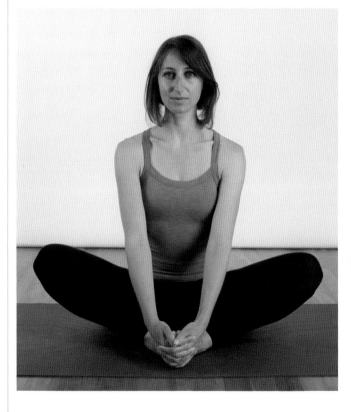

1 Begin this simple pose by bringing the soles of your feet together, knees bent to the sides, and heels drawn in close to the body.

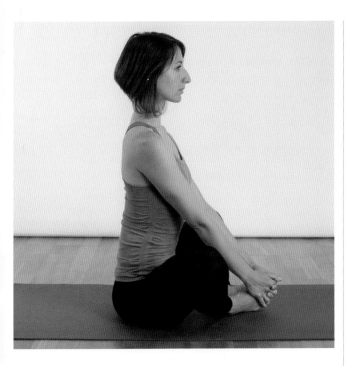

2 Clasp your hands around your toes, stretch your spine up, and take your knees down to the floor. Even if your knees are not on the floor, they should be level.

3 Stay in this pose for a minute or more.

Using Support
- Sitting on a pad or folded blanket makes it easier to lift the trunk and relax the hips, although you may then need to keep your hands on the floor behind your hips.
- Sitting with your back to a wall gives you more support and allows you to stay longer in the posture without strain.

Upavistha Konasana—Seated Angle Pose

There is a pronounced wide angle between the legs in this sitting position and forward bend. It is a pose that stretches the hamstrings and can relieve sciatica.

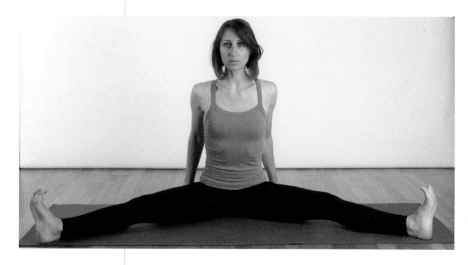

1 Sit up straight and take your legs very wide apart. Your feet should be upright so the center of the back of each heel is on the floor and your kneecaps face the ceiling. Keep your legs straight, with the backs of your thighs pressing down. Placing your hands on the floor behind your hips for support, lift your spine, and open your chest.

Using Support
- When sitting upright on a pad or folded blanket in the first stage of this pose, put your back against a wall to help it stay erect.
- If you find it difficult to reach your feet in the full or concave back versions of the pose, try using two belts, one around each foot.
- If you can go forward to the full pose easily, make the posture more relaxing by resting your head or the front of your trunk on a bolster.

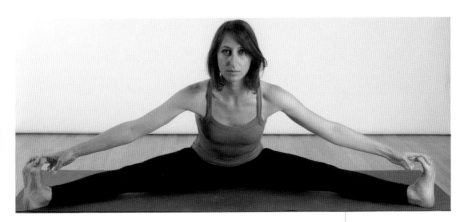

2 To continue into the forward bend, keep the extension in your spine, exhale, and lean forward until you can catch your toes. Keep your head up and your back concave for a few moments, and check that your legs are still straight. This may be enough for you, since the back and inner thighs need to be very elastic to allow the full forward bend.

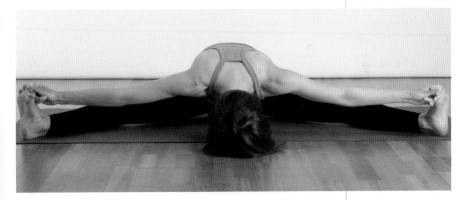

3 If you are able, continue the forward bend. Keep your spine extended and your buttock bones pressed firmly down. Make sure your feet are vertical. Do not let your legs roll in or lose the openness on the backs of your knees. Exhale and take your head to the floor in front of you, keeping the front of your body extended so your chest also goes downward and your spine remains straight.

Janusirsasana—Head-to-Knee Bend

In this pose, you bend forward and take your head onto or beyond your knee.

1 Sit in the Staff pose (see pages 68–9). Use folded blankets for support if your lower back does not easily come upright.

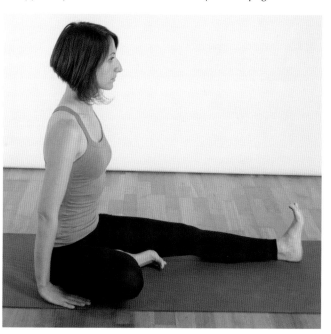

Caution
• As with other forward bending postures, do not strain the back or knees.
• If there is any pain in the lower back, sit on a support and use a belt, keeping the trunk straight.
• If the bent knee is stiff or painful, a support underneath it may help—or you may need to seek advice.

2 Bend your right knee to the side and draw the foot toward you, allowing the sole to turn upward. Place your right heel at the top of your right thigh. Keep your left leg extended, foot vertical, and draw up your trunk. Turn your chest and waist to face the straight leg, keeping the bent knee back.

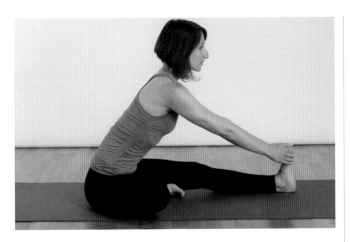

3 Exhale and lean forward over the extended leg, catching your left foot with both hands. Your left knee stays straight and your trunk stays turned to face the straight leg. Keeping your head up, lengthen the front and both sides of your body.

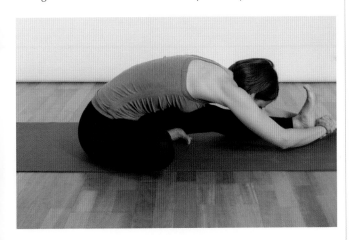

4 On another exhalation, stretch further forward and take your head down onto your shin. If you can take your trunk down on to your leg, you may be able to clasp your hands or catch your wrist beyond the foot. Make sure your shoulders stay level and let your back extend on both sides. Stay in the pose for about a minute. Repeat on the other side.

Using Support
• If you are able to take your head down, but not as far as your leg, it can be more relaxing to rest your head on a folded blanket or bolster placed on your shin.
• If you cannot catch your foot or if you have lower back problems, put a belt around the foot. Hold one end of the belt in each hand, with arms straight, and lift the front of the trunk. Keep your shoulders back and down, and check that they are level, as are your hands. Maintain the firmness of the straight leg.

85

Triang Mukhaikapada Pascimottanasana — One-Leg-Forward Bend

This posture is helpful for collapsed insteps, since both feet have to be active to maintain balance. Along with the other variations on forward bending, it is said to aid the health of the abdominal organs. As always, take special care of the bent knee and the lower back.

1 Sit in the Staff pose (see pages 68–9).

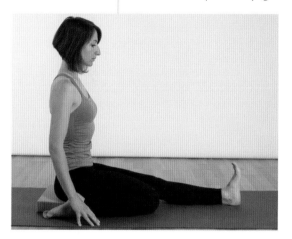

2 Bend your right knee and place your right foot next to your right hip, with the center of the front of your foot to the floor. Try to keep even your little toe down. Your left leg stays straight and your knees together. Stretch your trunk up, keeping both hips level.

3 Exhaling, lean forward, and catch your outstretched foot. Keep your head up and extend the front of your trunk. Stay for a couple of breaths, making sure you do not roll the weight over to the right.

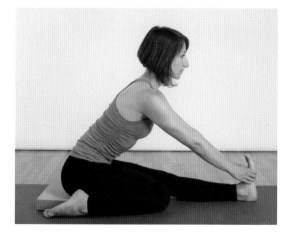

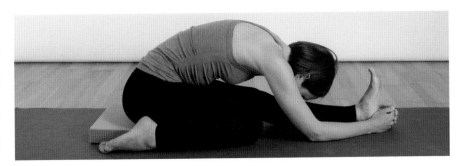

4 On another exhalation, stretch farther, and take your trunk down over your straight leg, head resting on your shin. You may be able to catch your wrist beyond your foot. Bend your elbows out to the sides to take you farther.

5 Stay in the posture, breathing evenly, for about 30 seconds, then inhale and come up to do the other side.

Using Support
The pose is more relaxing if you rest your head on a bolster or pad.

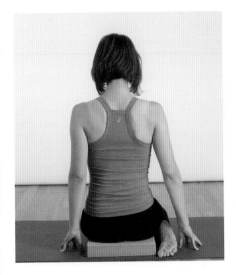

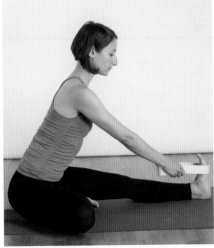

6 Your spine may lift better and you will feel supported if you sit on a foam block or folded blankets.

7 If you cannot catch your outstretched foot, use a belt to reduce the strain on your back and make the position more comfortable.

Malasana — The Garland

In the full Garland posture, you squat with feet together and knees apart, widen the knees, and take the trunk down so that the head goes to the floor. The arms then stretch back under the shins and up around the outsides of the upper thighs to catch hands behind the waist. It is this twining and linking of the arms that gives the pose the name of Garland (Malasana in Sanskrit). Mala also means a rosary, a string of beads, used for counting and focusing the mind in meditation. Although the full posture is difficult, the preparatory version shown here is beneficial. It brings flexibility to hips and ankles and can relieve lower backache during menstruation. Do not persist if the position hurts your knees.

Caution
Occasionally, people feel dizzy if they stand up too quickly from the Garland pose, so be careful. If you have felt dizzy coming up from this posture before, go into a sitting position and straighten your legs for a few moments before standing up.

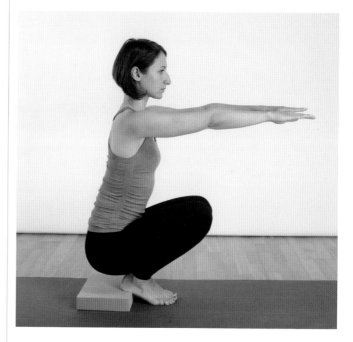

1 Squat with your feet joined together from heels to big toes. Your buttocks stay off the floor, but keep them low so there is no gap between thighs and calf muscles. Keep your heels down.

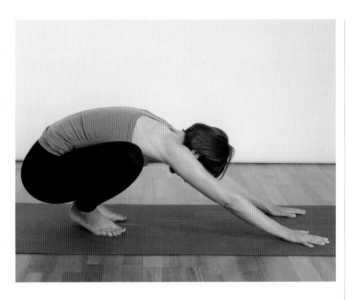

2 Separate your knees, and take your trunk forward and down between your thighs. Stretch your arms forward and relax your head toward the floor. Alternatively, you can take your arms back under your shins and clasp the back of your ankles.

3 Stay for up to a minute, then raise your head, and sit down or stand up.

Using Support
- If you cannot take your heels to the floor, support them on the edge of a folded blanket or pad.
- To make the pose more relaxing, rest your head on a support.
- If you cannot manage at first to squat with your feet together, let them be apart or turn your toes out slightly.
- Do not let your knees collapse inward, however—they should stay as wide apart as your toes are .
- Using a wall to support your lower back means you can try the pose with your heels down, without worrying about falling over backward.

Marichyasana—Maricy's Pose I

This posture is named after Maricy, one of the "seven celestial sages" of Indian mythology. The first stages can be done on their own; their emphasis is on twisting the trunk and starting to improve flexibility in the hips and shoulders. The full pose is a forward-bending variation, which tones the abdominal organs and helps to prepare for full forward bending.

1 Sit in the Staff pose. It is easier to do the posture well if you sit on a folded blanket or pad.

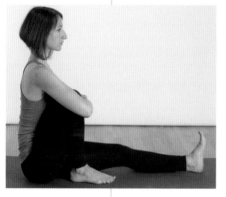

2 Bend your right knee up, bringing your right heel in close to the back of the inner right thigh. Your left leg stays straight, with your foot vertical. Stretch your spine up.

3 Turn your trunk to the left, placing your left hand behind you, and your right arm against the inside of your right knee to help you turn.

Caution
If you have had any lower back pain or problems in the past, be very careful when attempting this pose. Take your time and ease gently into the posture.

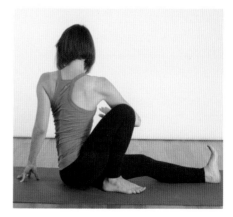

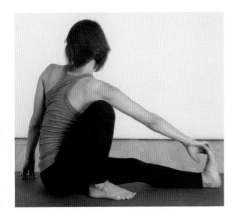

4 Lean the right side of your trunk toward your right leg and extend your right arm toward your outstretched foot, still turned to face the left.

5 With your inner right thigh against your outer right side of your back, turn your right arm inward so that the thumb points down.

6 Bend your right arm around the bent leg and bring your hand around behind your back to catch your left wrist if you can (use a belt to make a connection if necessary). This is the twisting posture. Your chest should remain lifted.

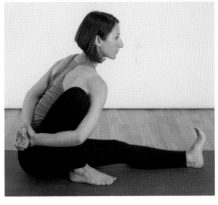

7 To continue into the forward bend, still clasping hands, turn your trunk back to face the straight leg. Exhale and bend forward, taking your head to your left shin if possible. The left side of your waist has to come forward toward the straight leg so both shoulders can be on the same level.

8 Stay in the pose for 20–30 seconds. Then inhale, come up, release your hands, and repeat on the other side.

91

Marichyasana — Maricy's Pose III

This is another twisting posture dedicated to the sage Maricy. The full posture, sitting on the floor, calls for mobility in the shoulders. This pose, like all the twisting postures, can help to strengthen the back and restore its flexibility.

Sitting Twist

The intense Seated Twist is said to have a beneficial effect on the digestive system as well as the back—provided, of course, that you do not do it soon after eating!

1 Sit in the Staff pose (see pages 68–9). Using a pad or folded blanket gives you a better lift of the trunk and hence easier twisting.

2 Bend up your right knee and place the foot on the floor with your heel close to the groin. Stretch up your spine.

3 Exhale, turn your trunk to the right, and place your right hand on the floor behind you. If you would have to lean back to reach the floor, put your hand on a support or against a wall. Take your left arm to the outside of your right thigh, and press the arm against your leg to help you turn more. Keep your left leg straight and your right shin upright, resisting the push of your left arm. As you turn, continue stretching your spine.

4 Stay in the posture, breathing evenly, for about 30 seconds, then repeat on the other side.

Standing Twist

An easier, standing version of this pose can be achieved by following these basic steps with a standard household chair as a prop.

1 Take a sturdy chair or stool and place it next to a wall. Stand facing it in the Mountain pose (see pages 44–5), with the wall next to your right side.

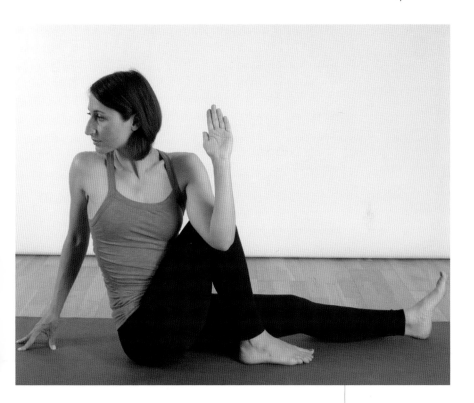

2 Lift your right leg and place the sole of that foot on the stool, keeping the knee bent up. Your left leg stays stretching up and both feet face forward.

3 Stretch your trunk up and turn to face the wall, keeping your shoulders level. Place your right hand on the wall and your left hand on your bent knee to help you turn. Do not push the bent leg over, but keep it near the wall. Your left leg and your trunk should remain upright and extended.

4 Stay for about 30 seconds, then repeat, with the wall on your left and your left leg on the chair.

Bharadvajasana I – Bharadvaja's Pose I

This posture—Bharadvajasana I—is named after Bharadvaja, a mythical sage. You can do the pose most easily sitting on a chair. When it is done on the floor, sitting on a blanket helps the trunk to stretch up evenly.

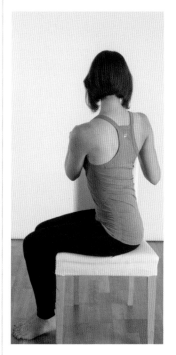 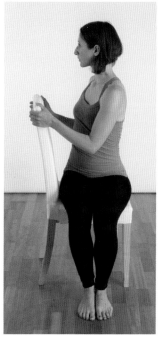

Bharadvajasana I on a Chair

1 Sit sideways on a chair with your legs together and your feet flat on the floor and your knees at right angles.

2 Stretch up your spine and turn to the right, using your hands to help increase the twist. Your trunk should stay vertical, your shoulders level, and there should be no strain in your neck.

3 Stay for about 30 seconds, then repeat, twisting the other way.

Bharadvajasana I on the Floor

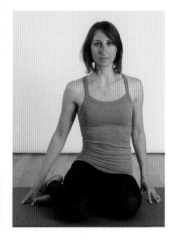 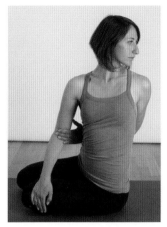

1 Sit in the Staff pose (see pages 68–9). Bend both legs and take them to the right side, with your right ankle on top of your left instep. Keep your knees and hips down and stretch your spine up.

2 Turn your trunk to the right, with your right hand on the floor behind you and your left hand on the outside of your chest to help you turn. Keep your shoulders level and your spine extended upward, chest open. Stay in this position for about 30 seconds on each side, or continue to the full pose.

3 While twisting, bend your left arm behind your back and catch your right upper arm. You may have to bend your right elbow to do this. Place the back of your right hand against the outside of your left thigh, and straighten your right arm. This turns you even farther in the pose. Stay for about 30 seconds, then repeat on the other side.

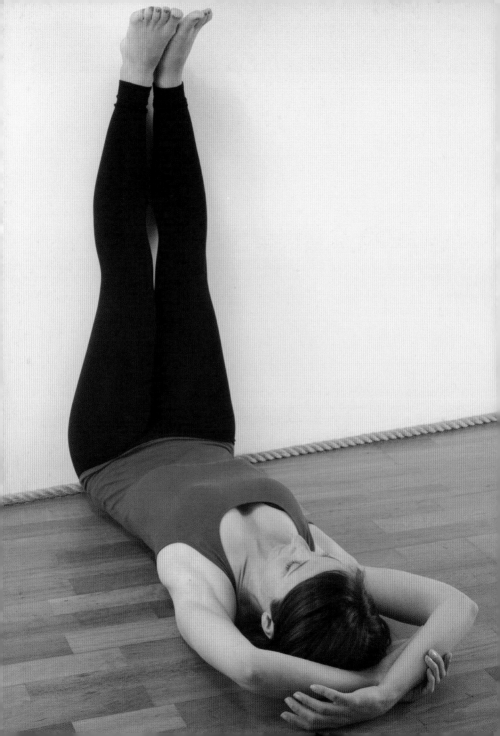

Supine Postures

Lying-down (supine) postures are the least physically tiring, so you can hold them for longer with a tranquil frame of mind. Upside-down (inverted) postures can be harder initially, but they have a refreshing effect and can be held for several minutes. Some of the positions can be intense stretches; the extra time spent in them allows for the gradual release of tension and lengthening of muscles. Other poses are comfortable and restful; for these, the longer timing is welcome and allows deeper relaxation. One word of caution: inverted poses are definitely not recommended at any stage of pregnancy or during menstruation.

Supta Virasana—Reclining Hero

In the reclining version of the Hero, the fronts of your hips open more, while your back is supported and your legs can rest. This posture has a calming and refreshing effect. It stretches the front of the body and gives relief to tired legs. Most people will need support to make the pose comfortable and safe. Do not persist if there is pain in the knees or back.

1 Sit between your feet in full Hero pose (see pages 72–3). Follow the instructions for the supported version, but do not use a pad to sit on. To lie back, you must be able to take your bottom to the floor without straining your knees. Sit evenly and stretch up your spine.

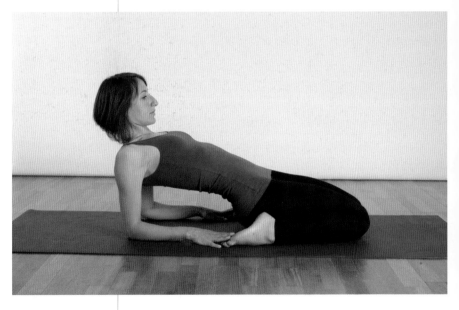

2 Lean back on your elbows, keeping your waist extended, then lower your trunk to the floor and lie down. The back of your head, shoulders, and upper back should rest on the floor, with no pain in your knees or back. Your buttocks, knees, and toes should stay down, with your feet close to the outer hips.

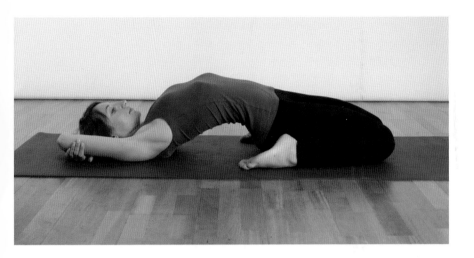

3 Stretch your arms along the floor over your head and stay for 30 seconds or longer.

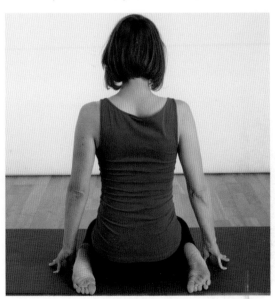

Using Support
Place a bolster or folded blankets under your back and head (which may need an extra blanket), but not under your bottom. Rest your arms by your sides and stay for a few minutes in the pose.

4 Use your arms to help you sit up again, keeping your waist long and your chest lifted.

99

Supta Baddha Konasana—Reclining Tailor

The Reclining Tailor is a restful posture for everyone, but is especially appreciated by women during menstruation, when it may relieve discomfort.

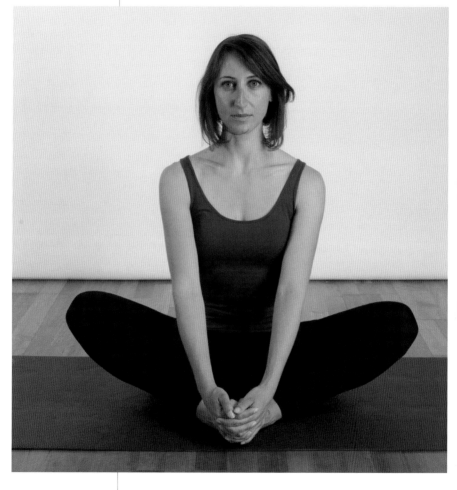

1 Sit in the Tailor pose (see pages 80–1), with your soles together and knees wide.

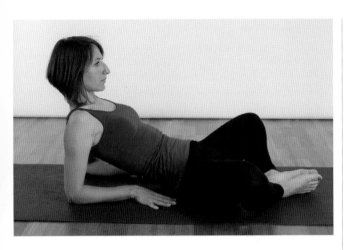

2 Keeping your feet close to your trunk, lie down on your back. Relax your legs and hips.

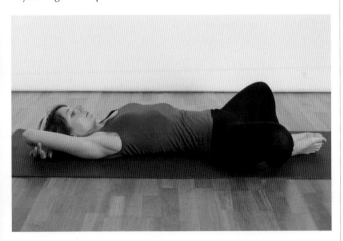

Using Support
• If your feet slide away, do the pose with your toes against a wall and bring your trunk close to your feet.

• If your back is stiff, place folded blankets on the floor behind you, so that they touch the back of your hips. Keeping your bottom on the floor, lie back on this support, arms by your sides.

• If it is hard to relax your hips, put equal support under each thigh using bolsters or rolled-up blankets.

3 Stretch your arms along the floor over your head. Relax the front and back of your trunk. Do not force your waist to the floor, nor deliberately hollow your back.

4 Stay comfortably in the pose for a few minutes. You can bring your knees together before sitting up again.

101

Bhujangasana — The Cobra

Postures in yoga are balanced. The Cobra mimics the snake rearing up, which gives the clue to its performance. It should seem a natural and inevitable movement, in no sense should it be straining for effect. In this way the front of the body is stretched; both chest and abdomen are opened up; the back and spine are compressed. A good way to start is to think of it as a slow, opening out dance movement, rather like the petals of a flower unfolding.

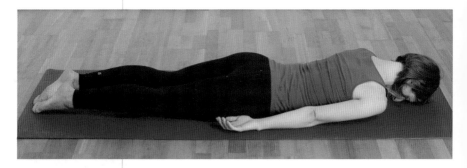

1 Lie face down on your mat with the heels and inner thighs touching. Your forehead should rest lightly on the mat.

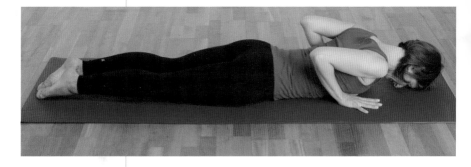

2 Place your hands underneath the shoulders so that the tops of your fingertips line up with the tips of your shoulders. Inhale a deep breath and lengthen your entire body through the sides of the waist and the crown of the head.

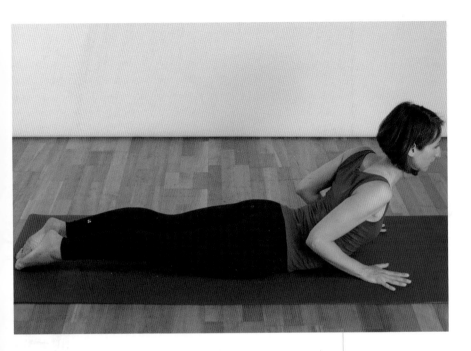

3 As you exhale, pull the inner thighs together so that the legs are active, and press down into the hip bones and lower abdomen to lift the head and chest off the floor. Keep the elbows tucked in to the sides of the ribs.

4 Maintain light even pressure through the palms of the hands but try to use the stomach and back muscles to support the pose rather than pushing through the arms too much. Press down through the tops of your toes; your feet should stay in contact with the mat throughout. Stay for 10–12 slow, deep breaths.

Variation
At first, don't hold the pose—instead, simply exhale to lift up and inhale to release back to the mat, until your back feels strong enough to hold the pose for longer.

Helpful Hint
As you progress in the pose, stop using your hands altogether; take them behind your back or out in front.

Salabasana — The Locust

Salabasana is a great pose to move on to after the Cobra (see pages 102–03). "Salabha" means locust, and the pose is so named because it resembles a locust at rest. This posture strengthens the lower back and abdominal muscles. The pressure on the stomach can help with digestive issues and is also said to be a stimulator of appetite. Best of all, the Locust has an invigorating effect on the body.

1 Lie face down as before, with your hands resting palms down alongside the body. Inhale to lengthen through the sides of the waist and crown of the head. Visualize your body getting longer.

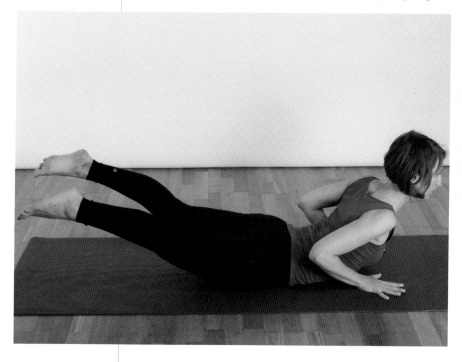

2 As you exhale, press down into the hips and lower abdomen and lift your head, chest and legs up into the air. Press down lightly into the palms of the hands. Keep the breath slow and even.

3 On an exhale, release the whole body back down to the floor and turn your head to one side.

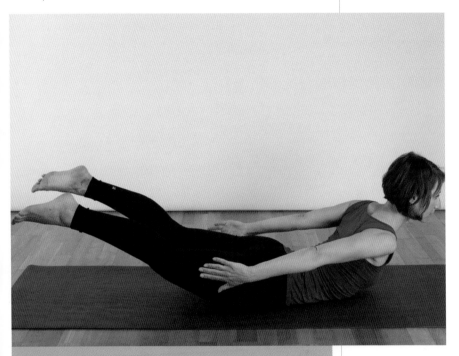

Variations

For a deeper bend, take the arms alongside the body with palms facing in toward each other. On an exhale, press down into the hips to lift as before while stretching your fingertips toward your feet and pulling your shoulders back and together.

Perform the pose with your arms in the air and with the fingers reaching back.

Abdominal Toning

In addition to creating a strong, flexible spine, the abdominal muscles must be kept in good condition. Natural abdominal control is essential for effective breathing and it also keeps the glands and organs in good shape.

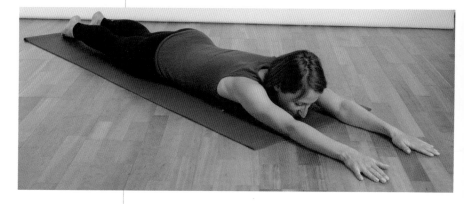

The Canoe

1 Lie on your front, chin against the floor, arms stretched in front, and with the feet close together.

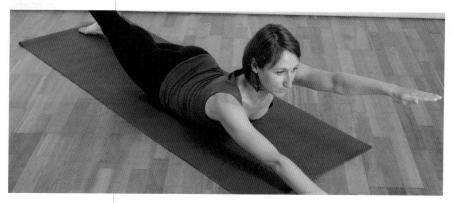

2 Having breathed out, stretch up the right arm and the left leg as you breathe in. Bring them down as you breathe out. Now repeat with the left arm and right leg. Perform each movement 3 times.

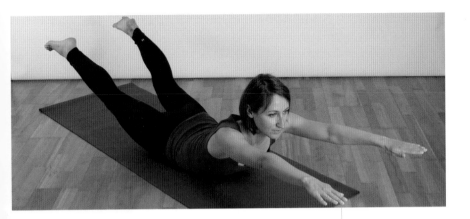

3 Finally, deepen the breathing a little and, as you breathe in, stretch up both arms and both legs, resting on the abdomen. Repeat this 3 times. Relax for a minute or two when you have finished.

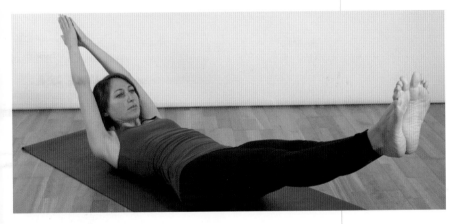

The Reverse Canoe

Lying on your back, feet together, stretch the arms on the floor over your head, bringing the palms together. After breathing out, breathe in and raise the arms, head, shoulders, and legs. Do not bring the hands or feet very far up from the floor—this will maximize the tension on the abdominal muscles. Breathe out as you come down, slowly. Repeat 3 times and then relax for a minute or two.

Supta Padangusthasana—Leg Stretching

The Sanskrit word "Padangustha" means "big toe." In the full sequence of this posture, you hold the big toe while stretching the legs and hips. It is hard to reach the toe at first, so use a belt to help you if necessary.

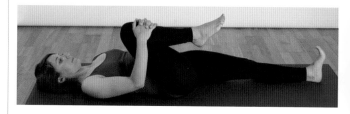

Stretching the Leg Up Forward

1 Lie evenly on your back, legs straight and together. Bend your right knee up toward your chest.

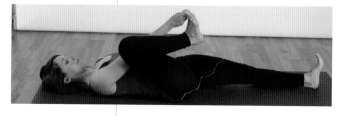

2 Catch your big toe with the first two fingers and thumb of your right hand. Place your left hand on the top of your left thigh.

3 Being careful not to disturb either your trunk or your head, straighten up your right leg. Your left leg presses down firmly with the left foot flexed. Keep both legs extended.

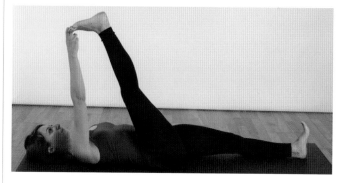

4 Stay in the pose for 30 seconds, breathing evenly. Then bend the lifted leg, release your hold on the foot, and repeat on the other side.

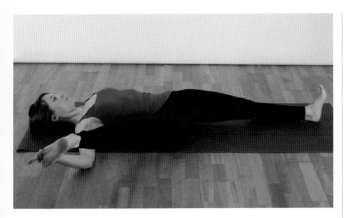

Stretching the Leg to the Side

1 Lie evenly on your back, legs straight and together. Raise and stretch your leg like with the Leg Up Forward position, holding your big toe.

2 Keep the left side of your trunk down, your left leg in line with it, left foot vertical, and lower your right leg out to the side. The leg should turn in the hip socket so that your right foot stays parallel to the floor. Take the outside of your right leg slowly down toward the floor or support, keeping both legs firmly straight.

3 Stay for 30 seconds or more, then repeat on the other side.

Using Support
- Use a belt if you cannot reach your toe.
- In addition to using a belt, you can press your bottom foot on the base of a wall. This helps to keep that foot upright and the thigh of the lower leg down. This can also be beneficial when you take your leg to the side, because the hips tend to tilt in the direction your raised leg is moving.
- The movement may be difficult to control even while pressing one foot against a wall. If so, place a block or a folded blanket under the foot or the top thigh of the leg that is stretching sideways.

109

Urdhva Prasarita Padasana—Legs Up Against a Wall

Raising the legs with support is a restful pose for everyone and provides a gentle stretch that is especially beneficial for those who are stiff or unable to work at more strenuous poses. In this posture, you hold your extended legs up vertically against a wall. You may be more comfortable lying on a mat or blanket, but make sure you do not slide away from the wall.

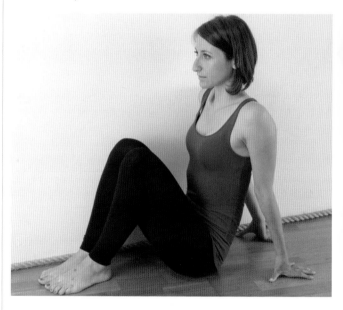

1 Sit with the wall touching your side, legs together, and knees bent.

Helpful Hints
- The posture can be more relaxing if, instead of stretching your arms, you rest them by your sides .
- If, when your arms are by your sides, the back of your neck shortens and your chin pokes up, place a support under your head so that your face remains level with the ground.

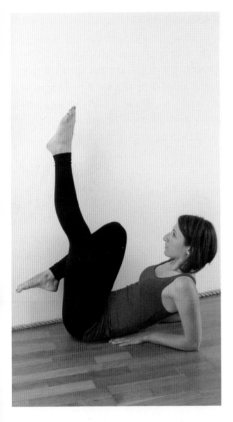
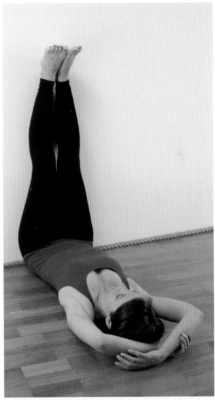

2 Lean back and swing your legs up. At the same time, move your trunk around so that it ends up perpendicular to the wall. Lie down with your bottom and legs in contact with the wall and your back and head on the floor.

3 Check that you are evenly positioned in relation to the wall and stretch your legs up. Relax the back and the front of your trunk, and take your arms over your head onto the floor. Stretch your arms and your spine, making sure you do not arch your neck.

Variation
You may have to make some adjustments to get close to the wall. If you are stiff and cannot achieve this, keep your back, hips, and head comfortably on the floor and let your hips be far enough from the wall to enable you to straighten your legs completely.

Setu Bandasana—The Bridge

This is a gentle version of the full Bridge pose, which is based on the Shoulder Stand (see pages 120–21). It can be wonderfully relaxing, and you can hold it for several minutes. Ultimately your hands on your back support the arch made by your body in the Bridge posture. On the opposite page, supports make the pose less demanding. Be careful to make sure your back does not feel constricted.

Unsupported Bridge

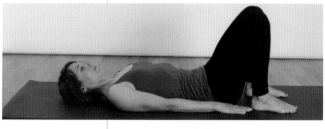

1 Lean back and bend your legs toward you, checking your position so that your shoulders and upper chest can come up easily from the mat.

2 Rest your shoulders and the back of your head on the mat, neck comfortably extended and chest open. Arrange your arms comfortably on the mat, bend your knees, and arch your back.

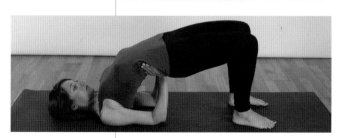

3 Raise your arms and support your back with your hands at the waist. After ten breaths, slowly come out of the pose by releasing the hands and lowering the spine and hips down onto the floor.

112

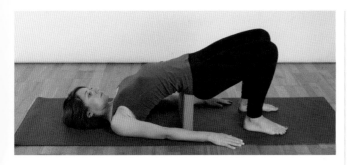

Using a Block for Support

If you are less flexible, you may be able to do the Bridge with a firm support under the sacrum.

1 Lean back and position yourself so the support is under your sacrum, with your pelvis high.

2 Rest the back of your head and your shoulders on the floor and your arms either near your sides or over your head.

3 To come out of the pose, bend your knees and push the blocks away so you can slide back down. Roll onto your side before rising.

Caution

The Bridge is a relatively advanced yoga posture that requires a significant degree of flexibility in order to be performed safely and satisfactorily. If you are in any doubt about the level of your personal fitness, and especially if you have suffered from back problems in the past, think carefully before attempting this quite demanding pose. If necessary, consult your doctor.

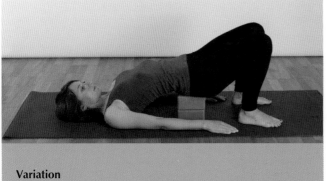

Variation

In the flexible variation, two blocks positioned carefully under your pelvis can replace the block used above.

113

Jathara Pari Vartanasana—Reclining Twist

Like other twists, the Reclining Twist can relieve backache. This is a gentle version of the full pose (which is done with straight legs); it should feel comfortable. Stop if you experience discomfort.

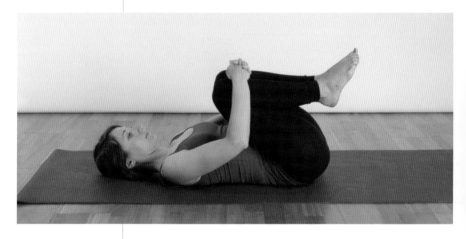

1 Lie on your back and bend your knees up to your chest.

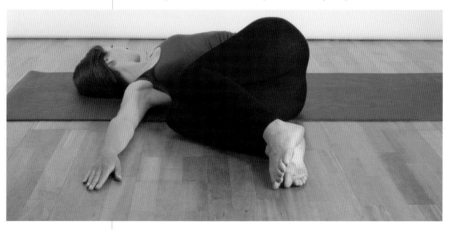

2 Keeping the acute angle between thighs and trunk if you can, lower your bent legs all the way to the ground on your right.

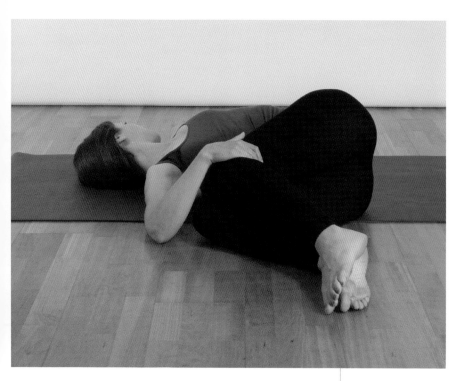

3 Turn your hips so you are lying on the outside of your right hip. Rest your right hand upon the outside of your right knee. Your left shoulder should stay down, but do not force it if it is painful, or if it stops your legs from going to the floor.

Helpful Hints
- Stretching out both arms, palms upward, helps to open the chest.
- If your legs tend to lift or slide away, hold them with your left hand.
- If stretching out the right arm is painful, let it bend—rest it on folded blankets if your shoulder is lifted far from the floor.

115

Viparita Karani—Raised Hips and Legs

In the Sanskrit name of this pose, "Viparita" means "inverted," and this is more of an upside-down than a lying-down posture. Its effects are related to those of the Shoulder Stand (see pages 118–19).

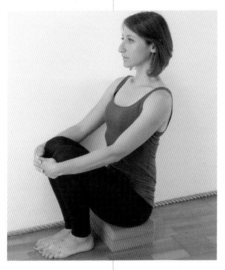

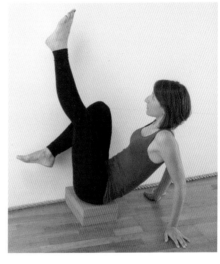

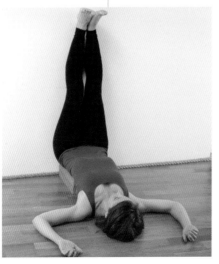

1 Place a block near a wall. The support needs to be higher and wider the taller you are. Sit on the support, sideways to the wall, knees bent.

2 Lean back and take your legs one at a time up the wall. As you do this, swing around to bring your trunk perpendicular to the wall, keeping your rear end close to it.

3 Keep the back of your hips and waist on the support and lie your head and shoulders on the floor. The legs rest together against the wall, and the arms can rest on the floor over the head.

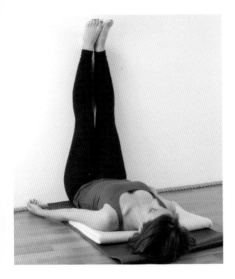

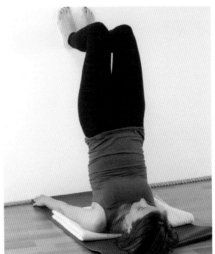

4 An alternative version of this pose can be done facing the wall head on.

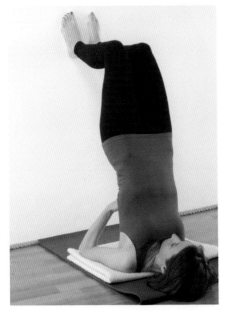

5 Press your feet firmly against the wall and push back, bending your knees, and taking the weight of your body on your shoulders, as they are forced down onto the mat. Stretch your arms out to your sides in order to control the posture.

6 Once you have settled in the posture and are feeling well balanced and in control, carefully bend your arms at the elbows, make your hands into fists, and push them into the small of your back, so as to support yourself in the pose. Hold for 30 seconds or so.

Caution
Like other inverted postures, this should not be done during either pregnancy or menstruation.

117

Sarvanganasana—Starter Shoulder Stand

This exercise follows on from Viparita Karani (see pages 116–17) and prepares you for the full Shoulder Stand (see pages 120–21). It can also help to overcome the difficulty of getting up into the pose.

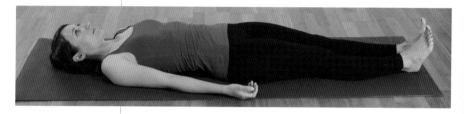

1 Lie calmly on your back on the mat and compose yourself.

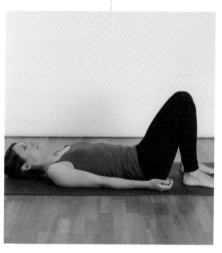

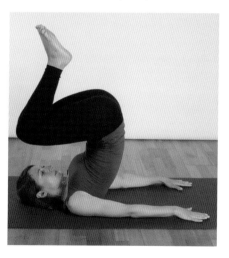

2 Bend your knees and draw your legs up toward you, keeping your back pressed firmly down on the mat with your arms fully extended at your sides.

3 Roll backward, taking the weight of your body on your shoulders. Bend at the waist so that your knees come down toward your face. Keep your arms fully extended at your sides and knees bent with your feet facing upward. When you are comfortable, move your hands to your back to support the pose.

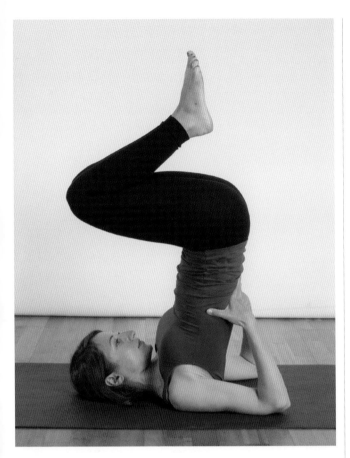

Caution
• If the posture hurts your neck, or if you experience pressure in the head, ears, eyes, or throat, come down and wait until you can get advice on how to do the pose safely.
• Do not perform this posture during menstruation.
• If you suffer from either high blood pressure or glaucoma, you should avoid inverted postures.
• Do not attempt this posture during pregnancy.

4 Open your chest and keep your elbows in. Raise your hips so your weight lifts off the back of the upper chest and more onto the tops of your shoulders. Place your hands on your back to add support to the upward stretch of the trunk, and straighten your legs. Keep your gaze on your feet to aid your balance in the pose.

5 Stay for a few minutes, breathing evenly. Then bend your knees and come down, using your legs to support you and control your descent until your back once more rests on the floor. Bend your knees and turn to the side to come up.

119

Sarvangasana — Shoulder Stand

This posture is sometimes referred to as the mother of the asanas, to indicate its importance. It works and affects the entire body— its Sanskrit name, Sarvangasana, means "whole body" or "all limbs" —and it has received considerable attention from medical research. Performed properly it has many beneficial effects, particularly on the metabolism and circulatory system.

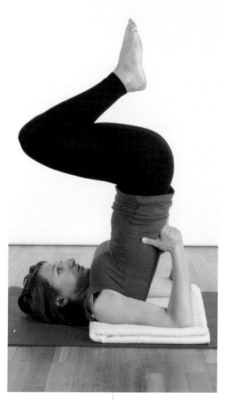

1 Lie on your back, with your head on the floor and your shoulders and upper body on folded blankets. Keep your arms close to your sides.

2 Bend your knees and bring your feet in close to your body. Check that you are straight: legs in line with your trunk, positioned in the center of the blanket, shoulders equidistant from its edge.

3 Bring your bent legs up and over your stomach and raise your trunk and hips. To do this, press your arms down and swing your legs up. Bend your elbows and place your hands on your back.

Using Support
- It is difficult to do the posture well on a flat surface. Blankets under your shoulders relieve any strain on your neck and make it easier to lift your trunk to a vertical position where your chest can be open.
- Fold the blankets neatly and evenly to give an area large enough to take the full width of your shoulders.

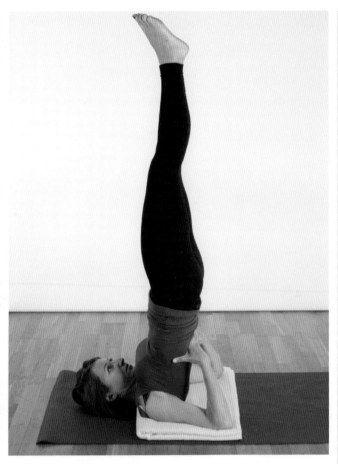

Helpful Hints
• Extending the height of the folded blankets under your hips makes it easier to come into and out of the pose.
• Your elbows should be shoulder-width apart to allow you to use your arms to help raise your back.

4 If you can, bring your hips higher, above your shoulders, and stretch your legs straight up. Use your hands to support your back in a vertical position, keeping your shoulders away from the ears, elbows down, and chest open. Bring your chest toward your chin and keep your neck and face relaxed.

5 Continuing to stretch your trunk and legs up, stay in the posture, breathing evenly. Come out of the pose by bending your knees and rolling back down, using your arms to help control your descent.

Halasana—The Plough

The Plough pose (Halasana) is normally done immediately after the Shoulder Stand (see pages 120–21), and its effects are similar. When taking the feet to the floor, you need to stretch the legs and back well; if you cannot keep your knees straight, use a support under the feet or legs.

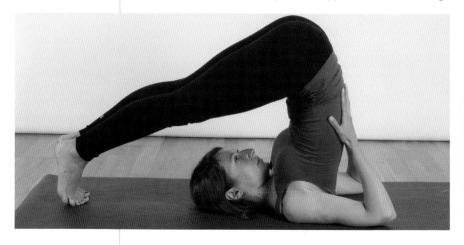

1 From the Shoulder Stand (see pages 120–21), take your toes to the floor (or onto a support), legs together over your head. If your back is weak, keep your legs bent as you lower them. Straighten your legs and raise your hips so the front of your body is extended as well as your back.

2 In the basic pose, your hands stay on your back. Lift your spine and extend your legs away from your trunk. Stay in the pose for 2–5 minutes without any strain in your head, neck, or breathing.

3 To release out of the pose, first bend your knees and bring them toward your forehead. Press your hands flat on the floor behind your back and press down firmly into the floor. Keeping the stomach muscles engaged, use your hands as brakes and roll down very slowly from the pose, rolling on to the back one vertebrae at a time. Do not roll quickly out of the pose and avoid jerky movements.

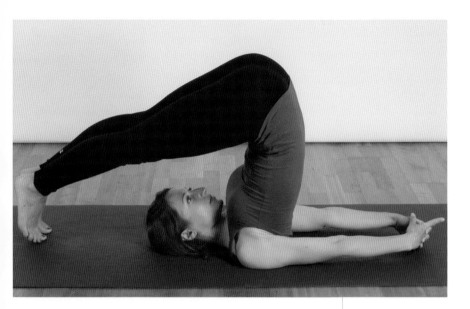

4 Once you become proficient at the supported version of the pose, you can try performing it without your hands behind your back. Adopt the supported pose in the same way as described on the opposite page and then simply lower your arms gently down to the floor, extending them fully behind you.

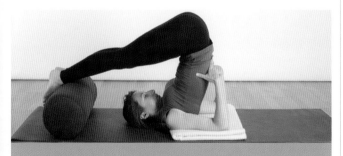

Caution
If you experience pressure in your head, pain in your neck or back, or difficulty breathing, take the feet onto a bolster. If this does not relieve discomfort, abandon the pose.

123

Matsyasana — The Fish

To counterbalance the deep neck stretch of the Shoulder Stand (see pages 120–21), we often go straight into Matseyasana to reopen the throat. Matseya means "fish" in Sanskrit. As in the Shoulder Stand, it is said to regulate the thyroid gland and boost the immune system.

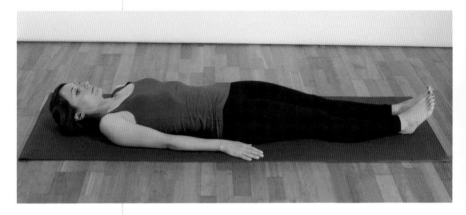

1 Lie flat on your back on the floor, arms resting by your sides.

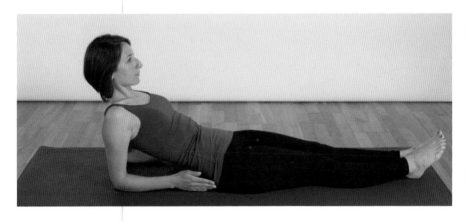

124

2 As you inhale, press down into the elbows, and lift the head and chest up off the floor. Keep looking down toward your toes.

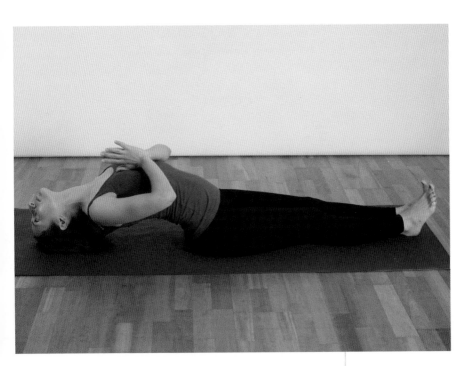

3 As you exhale, start to slide the elbows forward as you roll the top of the head down toward the floor. At the beginning, keep gentle pressure through the elbows to support the head and neck; eventually you hand-slide the arms all the way forward so you are balancing on the hips and the crown of the head. Draw the bottom jaw lightly toward the top jaw to open up the front of the throat.

Variation
Lie flat and take the hands behind the back of the head. Move the head back gently away from the feet and try to gain a sense of length through the front of the throat.

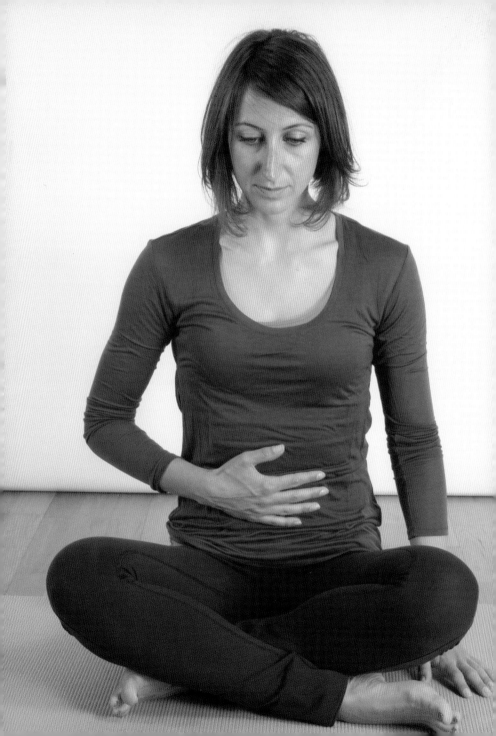

Relaxation and Breathing

Yoga can stimulate, strengthen, and channel the energy of mind as well as body. This chapter focuses on mental practice—the development of inner poise and serenity to match external balance and stability. Relaxing through yoga does not result in dull passivity, but in heightened clarity and sensitivity. Vigor is harnessed in quietness, where we can find freedom from the agitation that normally attends mental and physical pursuits. Breathing exercises control not just the passage of air but physical and mental energy. They show the way to greater inner awareness, concentration, and meditation.

Introduction to Relaxation

Yoga offers many positions that encourage muscular relaxation and a quiet state of consciousness. Several are lying-down postures, where much of the body weight is supported by the floor.

Below Sometimes, just lying peacefully on your back in a restful yoga pose is all you need in order to relax completely.

Sometimes relaxation is the result of intense stretching, when patience, careful effort, and concentration allow the release of physical and mental tension. Inverted poses can also have a refreshing and calming effect. When body, breathing, and mind are united in clarity and harmony, relaxation readily follows. At times when your body is tired or your back aches, it can be hard to work properly in physically demanding postures. Then, too, a simple, relaxing pose can be just what you need.

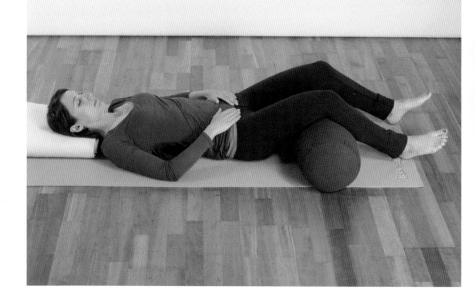

Savasana—The Corpse Pose

Sava means "a corpse," and Savasana is the pose in which the body lies motionless, as if dead. Even the breathing is slow and subtle, so it does not disturb the quietness of repose. With the stillness of the body and the barely discernible breathing comes stillness of the mind, although this takes perseverance to achieve. Practicing the posture improves your ability to release bodily tension and develop mental peace. Although you usually perform the Corpse pose in comfortable conditions, conducive to relaxation, you can also draw on the capacity to relax consciously in more stressful circumstances and completely change your prevailing mood and demeanor in the process. This is therefore a highly valuable pose and should normally be included at the end of each session. It gives you an opportunity to absorb and integrate the experience of your practice, removing fatigue, and refreshing body and mind.

Helpful Hint

As you first lie still, observe exactly how you are. If you notice something that needs correcting, adjust it promptly and quietly. Then rest completely, without any further disturbance.

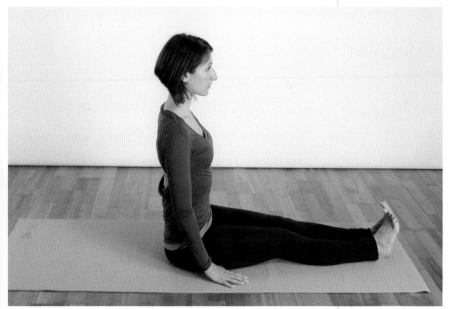

1 Sit in the Staff pose (see pages 68–9).

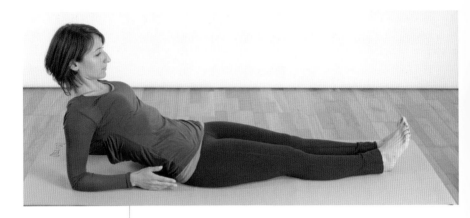

2 Lean back on your elbows and look down the length of your body to check that you are evenly positioned. Lie back so your neck does not overarch. Your neck and throat should be extended and soft.

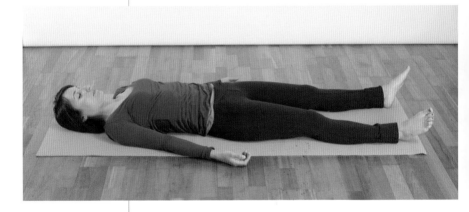

3 Stretch your arms and legs and turn your upper arms out so your palms turn upward and your shoulders stay down away from your ears; your arms should be placed a little way from the sides of your body. Relax your limbs completely, so your knees and elbows are not locked or stiff. Your feet and legs will roll away from each other slightly, and your body should feel comfortable. Close your eyes softly and relax your face, your head, and your whole body.

130

4 Take a few gentle, deep breaths, then let your breathing settle and become slow, quiet, and even. There should be no strain in the breathing and no awkwardness in the body's position. Stay for 5–15 minutes, breathing evenly, relaxing your body, and allowing your mind to become quiet.

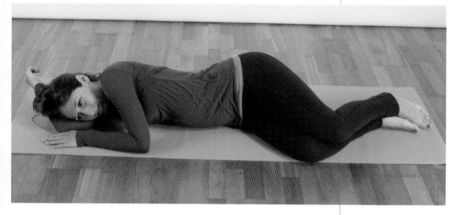

5 When you finish, do not stand up abruptly. Open your eyes without moving your gaze around, bend your knees, turn and lie on your right side for a little while. If you have been resting profoundly or for a long time, then stay in this position for a while longer and do not rush to get up.

The Right Conditions
- Before you start, anticipate what will make it easier for you to relax with alertness.
- Do not choose an uneven or drafty place in which to practice this posture.
- Make sure that you will be warm enough, but avoid restricting your body with bulky or tight clothing or heavy coverings.
- Lie on a surface that offers some padding but is not so soft that you sink into it.

Resting With Legs On a Chair

In this variant of the Corpse pose (see pages 129–31) the lower legs are supported on a chair. This is particularly restful for the back.

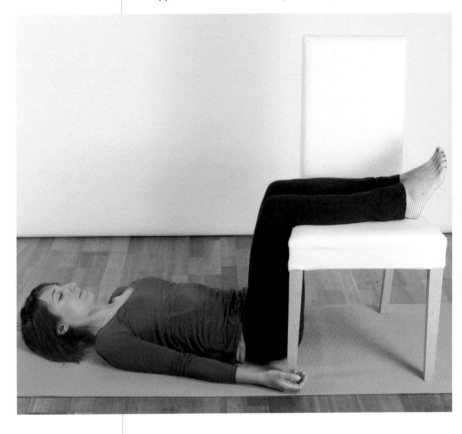

1 Find a level chair or stool of suitable height—pad a seat that slopes or is too low.

2 Lie on your back with a folded blanket under your head, bend and lift your legs, and rest your lower legs on the seat of the chair.

3 Close your eyes and breathe evenly. Rest for several minutes, then take your legs off the chair and turn to your right side before getting up.

Total Relaxation

In the Corpse pose, let your body be still and allow your breathing to take place naturally. Observe how you are positioned, and notice the contact between your body and the surface you are lying on.

- Release tension from the back of your body and then the front. Without physical disturbance, recognize mentally the places where tension remains.
- Relax the back of your trunk, from hips to shoulders, so it does not contract sideways or lengthwise.
- Relax the entire front of your trunk, including your abdomen and your chest.
- Relax your feet—the soles, the toes, the tops of your feet—and your legs, letting the muscles become soft and passive.
- Relax your arms and your hands, letting your fingers curl gently and your palms stay soft.
- Release tension in your neck and throat.
- Relax your scalp, the hairline area, and your temples, and let the skin of your face soften and relax.
- Close your eyes by bringing the upper lids down gently to meet the lower lids, keeping your eyeballs still and your brow relaxed.
- Let your tongue rest on the lower palate, teeth parted slightly so your jaw is not clenched.
- If you find it impossible to release tension in a particular area, do not dwell on this difficulty, but let go mentally and relax the rest of your body.
- Allow your breathing to continue quietly, stilling your mind to match the stillness of the pose.

After Your Practice

- Different postures have quite different effects; you may feel rested and peaceful or energized and alert. Try to observe these results and then match your choice of postures to your needs.
- Avoid rushing around or plunging into vigorous activity immediately after your practice.
- Wait about half an hour before eating, if possible.

When it Doesn't Work

Sometimes the mind and body remain agitated or tense, despite your best efforts to relax. Other times, you may fall asleep. In these cases, accept that full relaxation with awareness has eluded you—but do not be discouraged. This is one of the hardest yoga skills to learn.

133

Introduction to Breathing

Even with assiduous practice of yoga postures, it is difficult to attain peace of mind if your thoughts and emotions are in turmoil. It is the combination of the postures (asanas) with breathing exercises (Pranayama) that helps develop a healthy body and mind.

R elaxation means release from cares, or rest, and implies a physical and a psychological lessening of tension. Exercises for the body, together with breathing, can help you learn to dispel unnecessary muscular tension and direct your energy appropriately. A moderate lifestyle and a healthy diet make it easier. Allowing your thoughts and actions to be guided by wisdom and compassion can bring benefits that will be felt by you and by others.

Even when you pay it no particular attention, your breathing responds to different positions of your body. If you are able to concentrate and attend to your breathing, as well as to the other aspects of a posture, your practice is intensified, and its effects can be felt more strongly. This sort of focused concentration is an essential preparation for meditation (see pages 176–85). Classical meditation positions, such as the Lotus pose (Padmasana) (see pages 154–57), are well known, but every yoga posture is potentially a posture of meditation. Sustaining the relaxed alertness necessary for meditation, however, is easier in some poses than in others. Similarly, control of the breath is more readily achieved in certain positions. Breathing continues as you hold the poses (the few practices where the breath is held are not covered here). Each posture affects the way you breathe, and many directly encourage more effective respiration by opening the chest, strengthening the abdomen, or releasing tension in the diaphragm.

Control of the breath and of the mind start with awareness of their activities. It is easiest to achieve this when those activities are simple, so the first exercise here places the body in a relaxing position while you watch yourself breathing normally.

134

Supported Corpse Pose

This pose is a variation of the Corpse pose (see pages 129–31) that opens the chest through the use of additional support under the back and head, allowing easier breathing and relaxation.

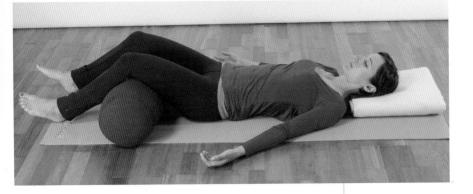

- Fold blankets neatly to support the length of your back and head. They should not be too wide or they will get in the way of your arms and hinder the opening of the chest. Place another blanket where your head will rest. Tuck a bolster underneath your knees.

- Sit in front of the pile of blankets with one of its narrow ends behind your hips, and lean back. Extend the back of your neck comfortably without tightening your throat. Stretch your legs and arms, turning the upper arms outward, a little away from your sides.

- Relax all your limbs, your hands, and your feet. Let your whole body rest comfortably and close your eyes. Relax your face and let your breathing settle naturally to match the stillness of your body.

Observing Your Breath

- **Relaxing your breathing** To begin with, simply rest, releasing tension in your body. Be aware of how you are lying and let your weight sink into the floor and the blankets. As you lie quietly, it is natural for the breathing to become slower. Observe this, without causing your breathing to change.

135

Right Observation of the body or the breathing can also be carried out in an upright sitting or standing posture. It prepares you for exercises in breath control and can be used as a focus in meditation practice.

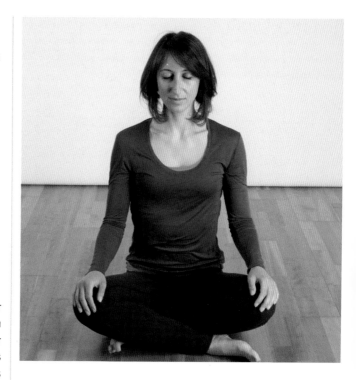

Releasing Tension

Tension may enter your body as you closely observe your breathing; notice this as well. Sometimes your shoulders and neck tighten, or tension creeps into your stomach, or your hands. Note the tension and release it, if you can, and return to watching your breath.

- **Sensing your breath** Notice through all your senses what happens on the inhalation and the exhalation. Feel the air as it enters and leaves your body through the nostrils—its temperature and other qualities. It may have a smell or a taste. Try to follow the passage of your breath within your body; even though you cannot feel where each molecule of air goes, you can observe how the different parts of your body react at each stage of the in- and out-breath.

- **Listening to your breathing** Although the sound of relaxed breathing should now be soft, you can still listen to the subtle difference between the sound of the inhalation and the exhalation. This inner listening helps to deepen relaxation farther. Keep your gaze turned downward, as though looking within your chest. This helps to keep your eyes quiet during your relaxation and to focus attention inward.

Resting the Head — Forward Bend, Cross-Legged

It is important to learn how to breathe well in all the different yoga postures. Resting the head as you bend forward is a good posture that allows the quietness to continue and you to concentrate on your breathing in an entirely different position. It is soothing to leave the head low and let the back stretch passively, but if your back is weak or your neck stiff, you may find it uncomfortable to lie flat immediately. This pose is good to do at other times, too, because of its generally relaxing effect.

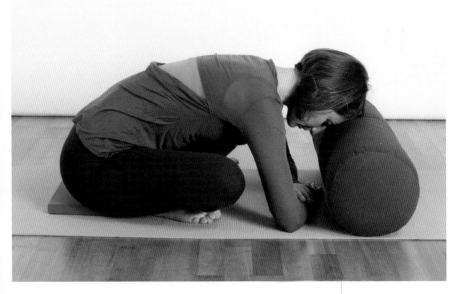

1 Sit in the Easy Cross-Legged pose (see pages 78–9). Sitting on a pad or a folded blanket will help by raising your hips.

2 Lean forward and rest your head on a support. This stretches your back and hips.

3 Rest in the Corpse pose (see pages 129–31) to finish, remembering to move your trunk off the folded blankets (they may be convenient to rest your head on).

137

Enhancing the Breath

The bottom ribs play a decisive role in breathing. Bad posture and agitated thoughts damage the breathing process, but with controlled breathing, the mind and body can be restored.

Sit or stand with the trunk upright. Do not overarch the spine. Become aware of your breath for a minute or two. Then begin to slow it down a little and ensure that it is rhythmical. Place the fingers lightly on the bottom ribs and become aware of their movement. The higher ribs play only a minor role and the abdomen is still. Concentrate quietly on the breath and its rhythmical movement. Be content to continue in this way for two or three minutes.

The diaphragm, attached to the bottom ribs, is dome-like, and when you breathe in the movement of the ribs stretches and partly straightens it. This helps the lungs to fill and also creates a vital pressure within the trunk.

Right Feel for your bottom ribs lightly with your fingertips and become aware of their position and importance as you relax and begin to control your breathing.

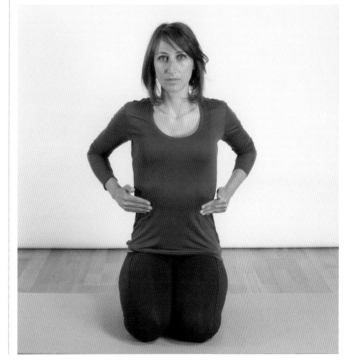

138

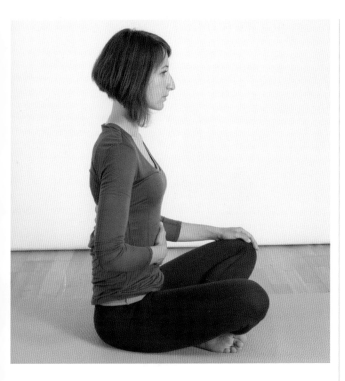

Left The bottom—or "floating"—ribs are designed to move up and out as we breathe. On the in-breath, muscles open these ribs; on the out-breath, they fall back. Sitting erect on a chair or on the floor, place the hands on the sides of the trunk, covering the bottom ribs. Breathe deeply and slowly and feel the ribs move. The chest and abdomen should be still.

As you breathe out, the dome becomes more pronounced again and the pressure is released. This is the essential stimulus both for energy and the natural functioning of the whole of the trunk.

You can enhance this natural breathing process and benefit from it accordingly. Lying down is useful, because it makes the process easier, but the same action can be carried out sitting erect.

Place the heels of the hands to the sides of the rib cage, against the bottom ribs. Concentrate on this area alone and, when you breathe in, let the ribs move out. As you begin to breathe out, firmly without jerking, press the ribs inward. If they are stiff, be careful but persist steadily. Only if a rib has recently been cracked or damaged is there likely to be any problem. The flexibility of these ribs is an important element of our energy, mental and physical. Continue the squeeze-and-release process for up to five minutes and then take the hands away and relax for a minute or two before getting up.

139

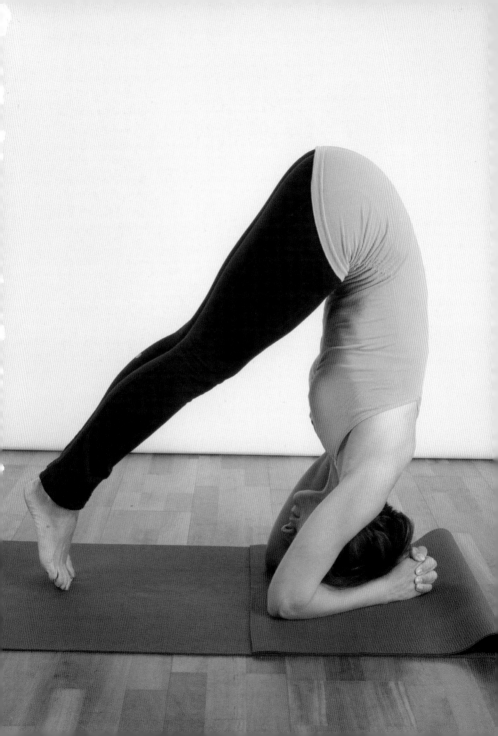

Advanced Postures

The postures in this chapter are more demanding than the previous poses. They require greater strength or flexibility, better coordination and balance, and deeper understanding of how the postures work with the body and mind. To safeguard yourself, check with a yoga teacher that you are doing them correctly. Even if you find some of the additional postures easy, do not neglect the more basic poses. They prepare the body for stretching farther and working harder. They teach discrimination and sensitivity, alongside the development of equanimity. One word of caution: advanced poses are not recommended at any stage of pregnancy or during menstruation.

Virabhadrasana III — Warrior III

This is a more advanced version of the basic Warrior I posture that can be found on pages 56–7.

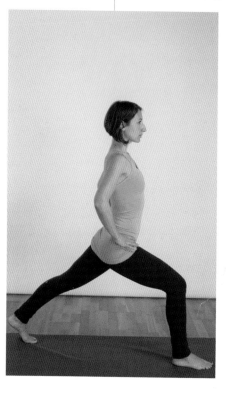 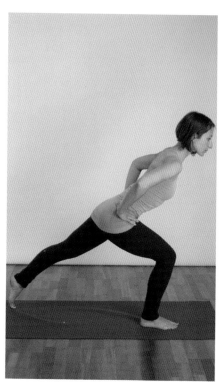

1 Stand in Warrior 1 (see pages 56–7). Exhale and bring your hands on to your hips. Inhale to lift through the chest and lift the back heel so that all 10 toes are facing towards the front of the mat.

2 On an exhale, start to bend deeply into the right knee and shift your weight forward onto the right leg. Pause with the very tips of the toes of the left foot still on the floor as you inhale. You will feel this very strongly in the right thigh.

142

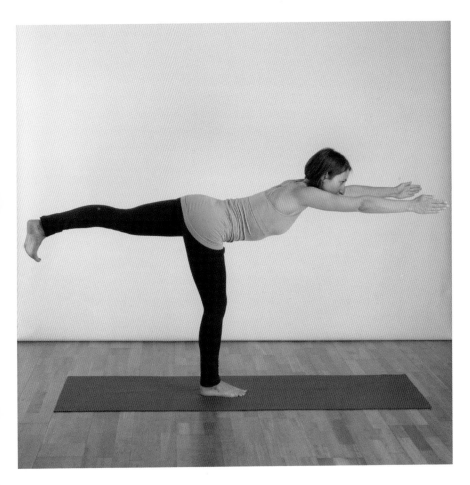

3 On your next exhale, keep moving your weight forward until you are balancing on your right leg. Flex the left toes strongly and keep the thigh muscles pulling onto the thigh bone. Imagine pressing out through the left heel and standing on the wall behind you.

4 Extend both arms forward, in line with your ears. Keep the neck and jaw soft and fix a soft gaze on the floor about a yard (one meter) away. Hold for 5 breaths and build up to 10 or 12.

5 To come down, bend the right knee and float the left toes back down to the floor until you are back in Warrior I. Step both feet to the front of the mat and repeat other side.

Ardha Chandrasana—The Half-Moon

This posture is named for its shape and for symbolic reasons. As light in the darkness, the moon represents illumination dispelling ignorance. The moon emits reflected light—a reminder that it is possible to draw on a source of energy and to shine without burning up. Despite demanding good control and mobility, this posture has a calming effect and can ease some back problems.

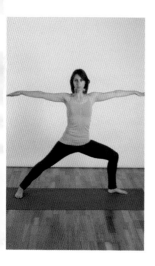 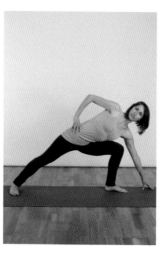 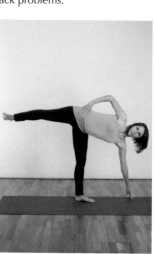

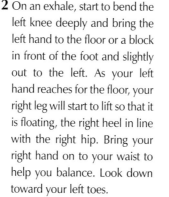

1 Stand in Warrior II (see pages 58–9).

2 On an exhale, start to bend the left knee deeply and bring the left hand to the floor or a block in front of the foot and slightly out to the left. As your left hand reaches for the floor, your right leg will start to lift so that it is floating, the right heel in line with the right hip. Bring your right hand on to your waist to help you balance. Look down toward your left toes.

3 Stack the right hip directly over the left and roll back slightly through the right ribcage so that the torso is facing straight out to the right and not down toward the floor. Flex the back toes strongly and pull the thigh muscle tightly onto the bone. The toes are facing out to your right as you press out through the back heel.

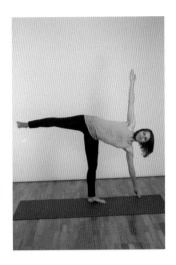
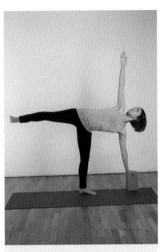

4 If you feel stable, raise the right hand straight up on an inhale. Finally, turn the eyes to look at the inside of the right palm. Hold for 5 breaths and then build up slowly to 10 or 12.

5 To come down, bend the left knee and float the right toes to the floor, finishing back in a Warrior II. Step the feet back together and repeat on the other side.

Helpful Hint

For a more advanced version of this pose, bring the left hand a few inches off the floor or onto your left ankle. Reach back and clasp the right ankle for the "sugarcane pose."

Using Support
- If balance is difficult, or the body goes out of line, practice this posture with your back against a wall. Keep your head, both shoulders, and your lifted foot on the wall, and your top hip, too, as much as you can. Your standing foot must be a few inches from the wall, but not so far away that your standing leg has to lean back. Keep your standing foot parallel to the wall.
- If your hamstrings are tight or your hips stiff, place your lower hand on a block (or a low chair), so the front of your body stays open and your legs straight.

Parivrtta Trikonasana — The Reverse Triangle

Not surprisingly, this Reverse Triangle stand has many similarities to the Triangle pose (see pages 52–3). However, the turn of the hips and twisting action of the spine make it a more demanding posture.

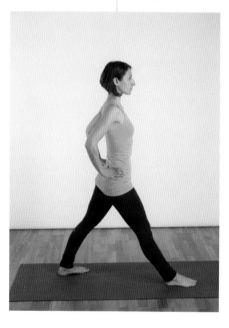

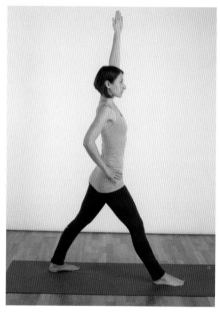

1 Stand in the Mountain pose (see pages 44–5). Jump or step your feet about three feet (one meter) apart, and check that they are in line. Stretch your arms horizontally to the sides, palms down.

2 Turn your left foot in about 45° and your right leg out fully to the right. At the same time, turn your hips and trunk to face the right. Keep your legs straight and stretch the spine up.

3 On an exhalation, continue turning your trunk to the right and take your left hand to the floor next to the outside of your right ankle. Keep the heel and outer edge of your left foot pressing down and your right big toe in firm contact with the floor. Stretch your legs and extend both sides of your waist.

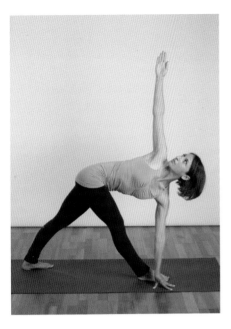 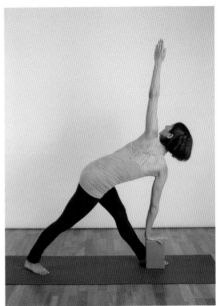

4 Stretch up the top arm so that both arms are vertical, and turn your head to look up. Continue to stretch your spine in the direction your right toes are facing, trunk revolving and chest open.

5 Stay in the pose for 20–30 seconds, breathing evenly. Inhale, come up and slowly untwist the spine to stand in Mountain Pose (see pages 44–5). Repeat on the other side.

Using Support
- It can be beneficial to do this pose even if you are unable to take your hand to the floor. Instead of reaching so low, take the hand to a block or low chair, placing it next to the opposite foot.
- You can also use a wall: put your back heel against it; or have the back against it when turned; or position yourself so you turn toward it and can place your top hand on it.

Sirsana — The Headstand

The Headstand, or Sirsana, is one of the most important practices of yoga and is known as the father of all the asanas, as the Shoulder Stand is the mother. The head, sirsa, is said to be the abode of the soul and the store of wisdom and understanding. When you stand upright, it is closest to the sun, source of light and power; when you stand on your head, it becomes your foundation. In the Headstand, intelligence and harmony should provide the basis of what you do.

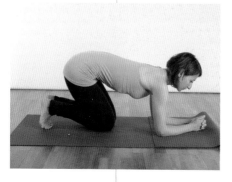

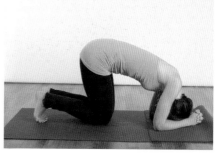

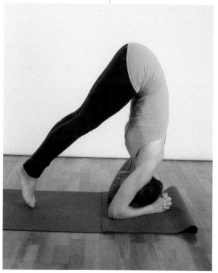

1 Take an evenly folded blanket and kneel in front of it, or fold your mat over as shown. Place your elbows on the blanket, no more than shoulder-width apart and level. Interlace your fingers securely and place your hands, thumbs uppermost, on the blanket, with your forearms, wrists, and hands pressing firmly down.

2 Put the top of your head on the floor evenly between your wrists, so that the back of your head touches the palms. Do not let your hands roll out.

3 Lift your hips and walk your feet in closer. Keep your shoulders spread and well lifted away from the floor and your neck long.

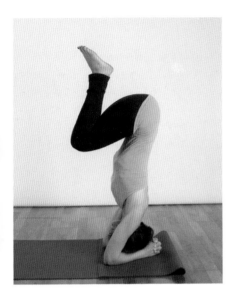
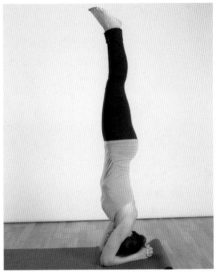

4 Raise your legs simultaneously and balance, not leaning to one side or the other.

5 Straighten your legs up together until they are vertical. Stretch your whole body up from the base, keeping the center of the top of your head on the floor and pressing down the outer edge of the forearms, from elbows to wrists. Keep lifting and widening your shoulders (but not your elbows), so there is no pain in your neck and no discomfort in your head. Ankles, hips, and neck should be in one vertical line and neither the lower ribs nor the tailbone should protrude.

6 Stay in the posture evenly and without strain for some minutes. Then bend your knees at the same time and lower your legs to the floor. Keep your head relaxed and down for a while before standing up.

Caution
All postures, however simple, can benefit from the help of an experienced teacher, but personal guidance is even more important for the additional poses, because incorrect practice can lead to injury. Don't attempt these postures during pregnancy or menstruation.

Uttanasana—Standing Forward Bend

This pose stretches the spine and legs. As you progress in the practice of yoga, you should deliberately seek to extend your understanding and awareness—an attitude expressed in the name of this pose. This pose, known as Uttanasana, indicates a deliberate and intense extension, but here it is performed as a relaxing pose. Although the legs are active, it has a calming effect and the back can fully relax.

Caution
• If you have back problems or cannot bend forward very far, do the supported version of this pose.
• Do not stay in a forward bend if you experience pain in the back, neck, or head.
• Even If you can bend easily, moving with the arms extended may put too much strain on your back. It is less demanding to come into and out of the pose with the hands on the hips first.

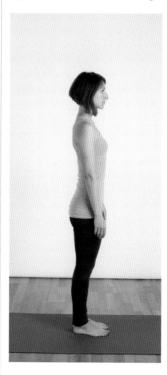
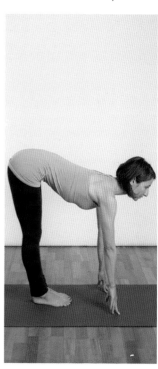

1 Stand in the Mountain pose (see pages 44–5). Your feet should be parallel, evenly weighted, and with soles and toes extended on the floor.

2 Exhaling, bend your trunk down, keeping your legs straight and lifting vertically. Relax your feet but draw up the front thigh muscles to support your knee joints.

150

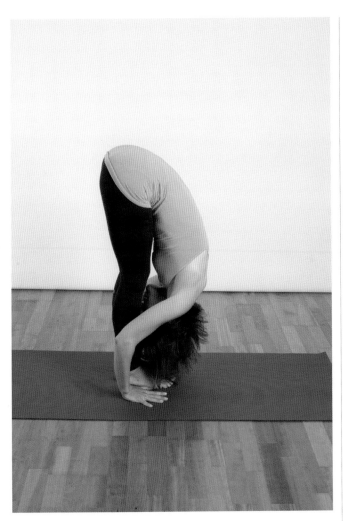

Using Support

• Choose a ledge that is at hip height (higher if you are stiff), and stand facing it with your feet parallel and hip-width apart .

• Place your hands on the ledge, leaning forward and adjusting the distance of your feet from the ledge so that your legs are vertical when your arms are straight .

• Keep your arms, hands and fingers extending and your legs strong—knees straight and front thigh muscles drawn up.

• Raise your head and lengthen the front of your trunk, then lower your head so that your ears are level with your arms. Keep the sides, front and back of your spine extending, so that your back does not sag or become rounded.

3 Place your hands on the floor and draw them slowly toward your feet. Relax your trunk, neck, and head, and breathe comfortably. Stay in the posture for 30–60 seconds. To come up, place your hands on your hips and raise your trunk, keeping the front and back of your spine long and the legs firm.

151

Navasana—The Boat

This posture owes its name to its shape. In Sanskrit it is called Navasana; nava means "a boat." Two variants are shown: paripurna "complete;" and ardha "half." Both strengthen the back and tone the abdominal organs, but Paripurna Navasana requires more flexibility; Ardha Navasana calls for strong stomach muscles. Do not persist with either posture if there is any pain in your back; however, do not give up if you shake a little and find them challenging!

Paripurna Navasana

1 Sit in the Staff pose (see pages 68–9).

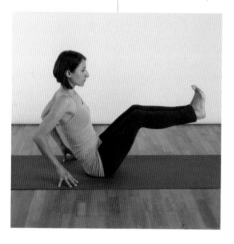 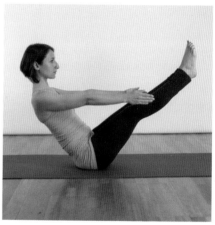

2 Lean back a little and balance with your feet off the floor. It is usually easier at first to bend your knees, but eventually you should come up into the pose with your legs straight and together.

3 Straighten your legs so your feet are higher than your head, and extend your arms horizontally forward, palms facing each other. Do not tip back past the base of your spine, but keep your chest lifted.

4 Stay in the pose for 10–20 seconds, breathing evenly.

Ardha Navasana

1 Sit in the Staff pose (see pages 38–9).

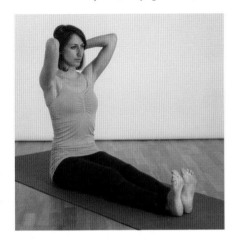

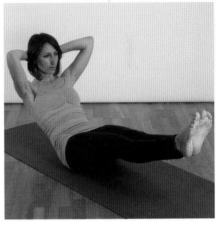

2 Interlace your fingers and place them behind your head, bringing your elbows slightly forward.

3 Lean back and raise your legs until they are about 30° from the floor and approximately level with your head. Keep them straight.

4 Stay in the posture for 10–20 seconds, while maintaining even breathing.

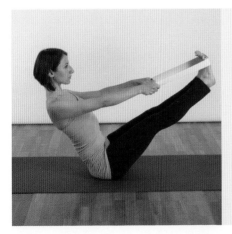

Using Support

At first it may be very difficult to maintain this V-shaped position for more than a few moments. Work on the balance and the stretch of the legs and spine by holding a belt around your feet. Be careful not to put additional strain on your spine by pulling on the belt too tightly; simply let the belt take the weight of your body in the gravitational pull of this posture.

Padmasana — The Lotus

Padmasana is one of the best-known yoga postures and is the classical posture of meditation. In much Eastern philosophy, the lotus symbolizes the human striving from ignorance and base concerns towards spiritual illumination.

Half-Lotus Forward Bend
This variation prepares you for both the full Lotus pose and forward bending. In Sanskrit it is called Ardha Baddha Padma Pascimottanasana.

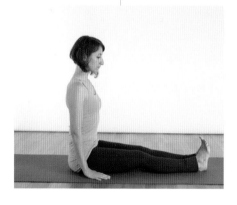

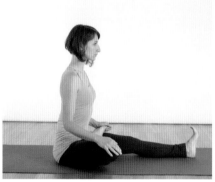

1 Sit in the Staff pose (see pages 38–9).

2 Bend your right leg and bring the foot high onto your left thigh, so that it touches your abdomen. Your right knee should face forward rather than to the side.

Caution
Folding the legs in the Lotus pose is difficult if the hips are stiff and can strain the knees, which are vulnerable joints. Do not force the legs into position if there is pain in the knees. An experienced teacher can tell you how to work safely toward the full pose.

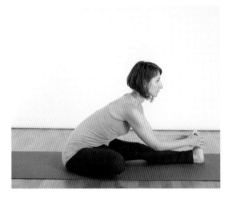 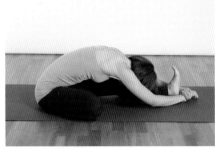

3 Bend forward and hold your left foot with both hands. Stretch your spine up, head raised and back concave.

4 On an exhalation, take your trunk down onto your straight leg and rest your face on the shin. Keep your left leg straight. Do not strain your back or the bent knee. Stay in the pose, breathing evenly, for 30 seconds or more, then inhale, come up, and repeat on the other side.

Using Support
- If you cannot easily reach the foot of your extended leg, or if you need to work with your back straight, use a belt around the foot of the extended leg.
- If your bent knee does not go down to the floor, support it with a block or folded blanket. This can be placed under the knee or under the ankle (where it can relieve strain in the ankle or foot).

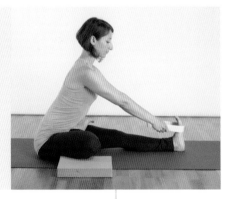

The Advanced Lotus

You may find that placing each foot on the opposite thigh is uncomfortable at first, but once learned, the Lotus position can become an ideal sitting posture for meditation and breathing practice, because it is stable and supports the upward stretch of the spine.

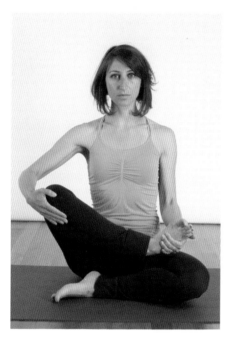 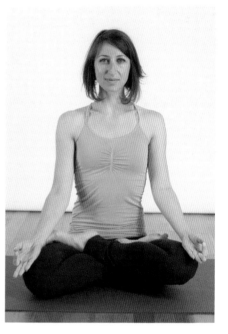

1 Sit cross-legged. Bring your right foot up onto the very top of your left thigh.

2 Bring your left foot forward, then lift it onto the very top of your right thigh, so your knees are near the floor and your soles face up. Keep your spine erect and stretch your trunk up, hands outstretched and facing upwards.

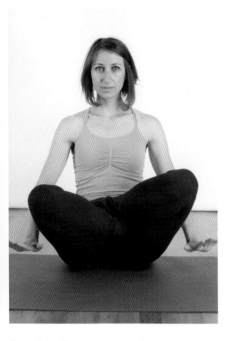

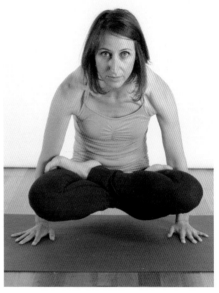

3 Rock back gently on your buttocks, placing your hands out to your sides for balance, pushing them down to the floor.

4 Carefully stabilize yourself, and then push down through your hands so that your entire body lifts off the floor, while retaining the full lotus position.

157

Eka Pada Raja Kapotasnana – The Pigeon

The Pigeon Pose is challenging, but well worth the effort. The thighs, groins, psoas, and muscles of the lower abdomen all get a really good stretch. When in the upright position, the open chest and shoulders form the pigeon's breast and the back leg represents the tail.

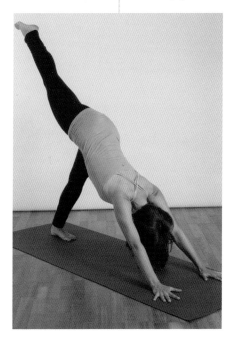

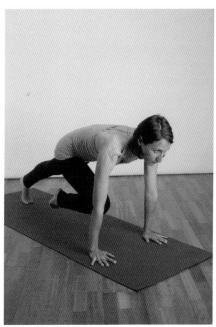

1 Start in a downward facing dog position. Inhale to lift the right leg straight up and back, keeping the leg engaged and the toes pointed. Press down into the heel of the left leg to feel a stretch in the calf muscle.

2 As you exhale, move forward into a plank pose and bend the right knee in toward the back of the right wrist.

Caution
You should not feel pain in the right knee. If you, do ease off immediately and place a yoga block underneath the right hip to ease the pressure off the front knee.

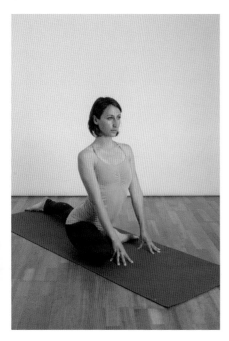

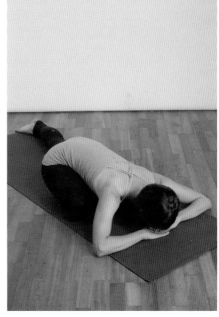

3 Drop the leg down to the floor. Look down; the shin bone should be diagonal to the top of the mat, with the tip of the knee slightly wider than the torso. Keep the hips level with the floor and try not to drop too heavily into the right hip. If the hip is floating, you can use a block to create support.

4 Press your fingertips into the floor and lift high through the crown of the head. Your shoulder blades will move back in space toward the heels. Keep lifting through the heart and chest so that the lower back remains open and spacious. The right hip will pull back energetically as the left hip moves forward.

5 On an exhale, start to fold over the right leg. Let the forehead come all the way down to the ground.

Variation

If the version with the forehead down is too hard to perform, prop yourself up on your elbows.

Wheel Preparation

Several of the more advanced yoga poses arch the spine backward. This is a movement that often becomes more difficult with age and can exacerbate back problems if not performed correctly. Refer to your teacher for advice about using support and how to practise.

Urdhva Mukha Svanasana—Head-Up Dog Pose
In this pose, the arms, legs, and back work strongly to lift the spine and open the chest.

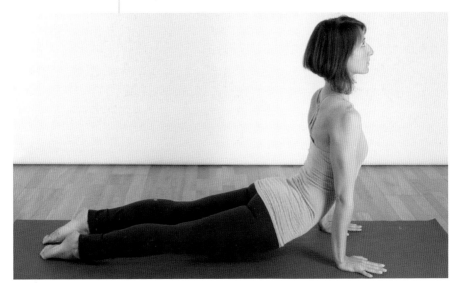

1 Lie on your front, feet slightly apart, and the fronts of your feet on the floor. Place your hands on the floor on each side of your lower chest.

2 Keep your legs stretching back and raise your head. Push your arms straight and raise your body up, with your straight legs staying off the floor (except the feet). Keep your hips low, tailbone tucked in, and bring your chest forwards and up between your arms. Stretch your spine up and take your shoulders back, making sure they do not hunch. Lengthen your neck and take your head back to look up. Stay in the posture for 20–30 seconds, breathing evenly.

Ustrasana—The Camel

The camel (ustra) is a creature that maintains a storehouse of energy even in inhospitable surroundings. This backbend can be done, under instruction, by relative beginners. It encourages mobility in the shoulders and an open chest.

Caution

Do not practice Camel pose if you have lower back or neck issues.

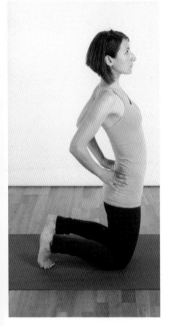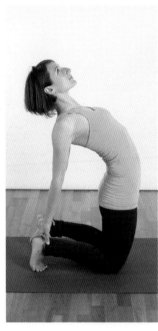

1 Kneel upright with legs together and thighs vertical. Place your hands evenly on your hips, with the thumbs near your lower spine, and stretch your trunk up.

2 Exhale, lift your ribcage, and arch back. Take your hands to your feet and keep your thighs stretched vertically. Lengthen your neck and take your head back. Keep your tailbone tucked in and forward and stretch your spine well.

3 Stay for 10–30 seconds, breathing normally, then replace your hands on your hips and come up.

Urdhva Dhanurasana—The Wheel/Upward Bow

In this pose, known as Urdhva Dhanurasana, the hands and feet push against the resistance of the floor to create an upward bow shape. It is the basis of the more difficult back bends and requires strength and flexibility. Practice of this posture has an energizing effect.

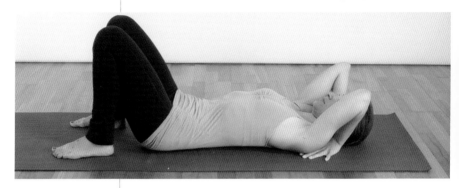

1 Lie on your back on the floor. Bend your knees up and place your feet close to your body, hip-width apart. Bend your arms and place your palms on the floor on each side of your neck, shoulder-width apart, fingers pointing toward your feet.

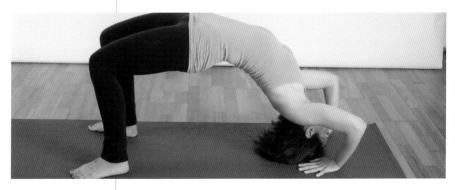

2 Exhaling, raise your hips and trunk, and come onto the top of your head. Keep your elbows in, so your arms are parallel to one another. Lift your tailbone.

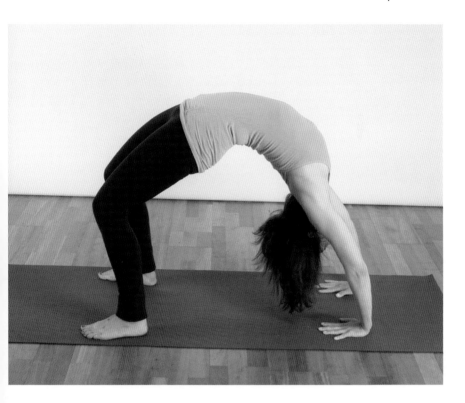

3 On another exhalation, push your hands and feet into the floor and lift your hips and trunk higher, so your head comes off the floor. Straighten your arms, open your chest, and stretch up your legs. You can raise your heels, bringing your feet in closer. Then keep the extra lift in your sacrum and the stretch on your abdomen as you replace your heels on the floor. Your feet should be parallel and all your limbs evenly positioned.

4 Stay for ten seconds or more, breathing evenly. Then bend your arms and legs and come down, tucking your chin in, so the back of your head can go to the floor as you lie down.

5 When you come down, take a moment to lie on the floor with the back flat, knees bent up toward the ceiling, and breathe into the lower back. After a while, bring the knees into the chest and give them a squeeze. Follow with some twists to stretch out the spine.

Bharadvajsana II — The Twist

The two twisting postures on these and pages 166–7 continue the work of Bharadvajasana I (see pages 94–5) and Maricyasana III (see pages 92–3). They both require greater flexibility in the hips and ankles. Take care not to strain your knees.

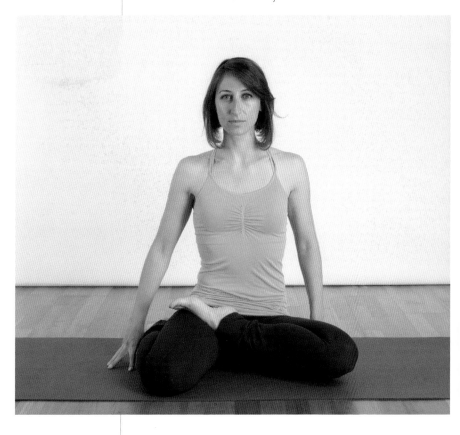

1 From sitting in the Staff pose (see pages 68–9), bend your right leg to bring the foot back next to your right hip (as in the full Hero pose, Virasana, see pages 72–3). Bend your left leg and place your left foot on top of your right thigh (as in the Lotus pose, Padmasana, see pages 154–5). Stretch your trunk up.

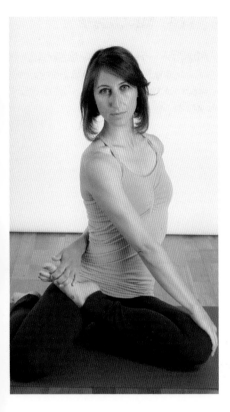
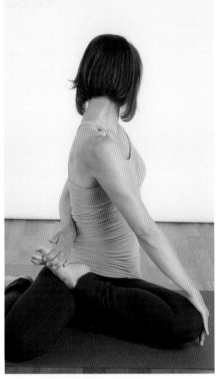

2 Exhaling, turn to the left and bring your left hand behind your back to catch your left foot. Place the back of your right hand against the outer left thigh.

3 Stay for about 30 seconds, breathing evenly, then release the foot and return to Staff pose. Repeat on the other side, twisting to the right.

Using Support
- Use a belt to catch your foot if your hand cannot reach it. Or work with your hand on the floor behind you.
- If your knees are stiff, sit on folded blankets or place one under the "Lotus" knee if that does not go down to the floor.

165

Ardha Matsyendrasana I—The Twist II

This is an easier version of the posture named after the earliest teacher of yoga. Legend relates that the deity Siva changed Matsyendra (lord of the fishes) from fish to human form because he had attended so closely to Siva's exposition of this pose.

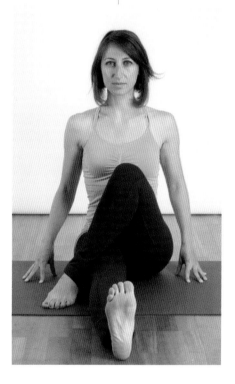 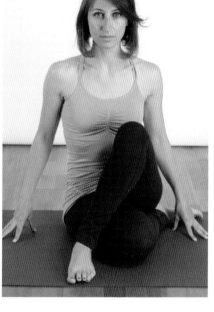

1 Bring your left foot to the outside edge of your right hip bone. The foot can come close to the body so that you can just feel the heel underneath the left hip.

2 Bend your left knee up and place your foot on the floor on the outside of your right thigh. Stretch up your trunk.

166

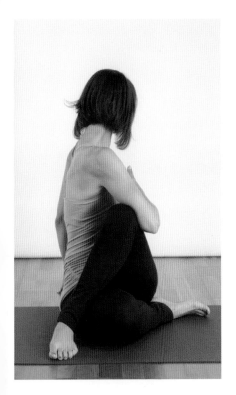
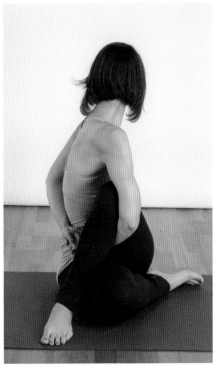

3 Turn to the left with your right arm onto the outside of your left leg and your left hand onto the floor behind you. Press your left arm against the leg to help you turn, keeping the left leg firm, shin upleft. You can stay here or continue to the next stage.

4 Closing the gap between the left side and left leg, bend your right arm around your left leg, palm facing out. Bring your left hand around your back so it can be caught by the right. Stay for about 30 seconds, then release and repeat to the right.

Using Support
- Sitting on your foot can be awkward and you may need padding underneath it or between your foot and your buttocks.
- Pushing against a wall or on a block can give a better lift and twist than working to catch hands or struggling to balance with your hand on the floor.

167

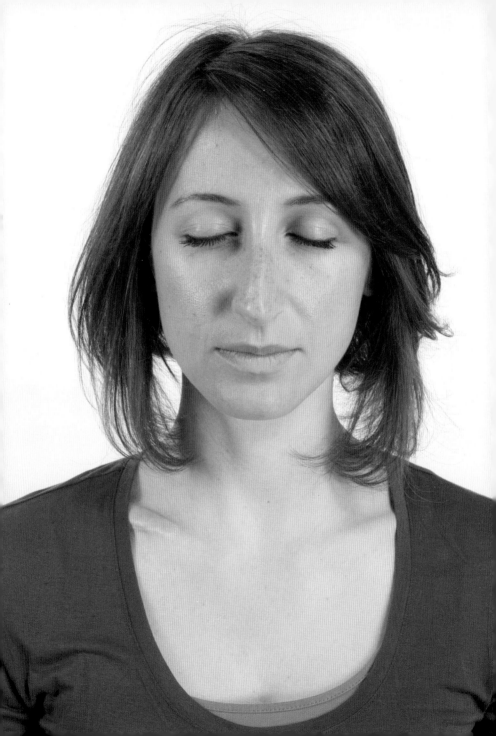

Mental Yoga

Yoga can be hugely beneficial in maintaining balance in your overall mental health. It helps you achieve deeper knowledge of yourself, which leads to self-acceptance. It facilitates in the discovery of your own power and makes you feel hopeful and optimistic about your life and general situation. Yoga practice can assist in calming the nervous system, which in turns helps to calm the mind and encourage clear thinking. Few forms of exercise are as good for you mentally as they are physically, but yoga is a rare case indeed.

Visualization

Visualization is a central aspect of human life; we conjure up pictures in our mind's eye all day long. Yoga trains us to take advantage of this natural phenomenon.

Opposite The best way to embrace visualization is to begin by emptying your mind. Imagine a perfect summer's day—a clear blue sky above a fresh green meadow, with just a few fluffy clouds floating across the horizon....

If applied with concentration, the mind has amazing strength. But, if you simply play about with the idea, results will be only intermittent and unsatisfactory. The ability to retain a simple mental picture can be one of the most important achievements of life. A celebrated Indian yogi, Swami Rama, was involved in experiments at the Menninger Institute in the United States, where he showed he could control the beat of his heart by visualization.

Swami Rama simply visualized a blue sky, with small, fluffy almost motionless clouds in it. Because his concentration was complete, the brain accepted this concept as reality and the whole body slowed down accordingly.

To visualize, you do not have to create an actual mental picture, but an impression; the feeling of the picture. Simply as an exercise, sit erect, close your eyes and imagine such a sky: a beautiful summer's day, just a few light clouds and the feeling of peace, warmth, and quiet. Beneath this tranquil skyscape lies a rolling green meadow, completely empty, with no one around. If other thoughts intrude, gently push them away. This can be repeated whenever you feel like it.

Controlling Thought

A well-known swami once declared: "Human beings will do anything to help themselves—except to work for it." Once you realize that visualization is a natural, built-in process, you can determine to make it a part of your life. Of course, the brain will keep interposing irrelevant thoughts, but as you persist this will happen less and less. Once you have gained substantial mental control, your life will be enhanced tremendously.

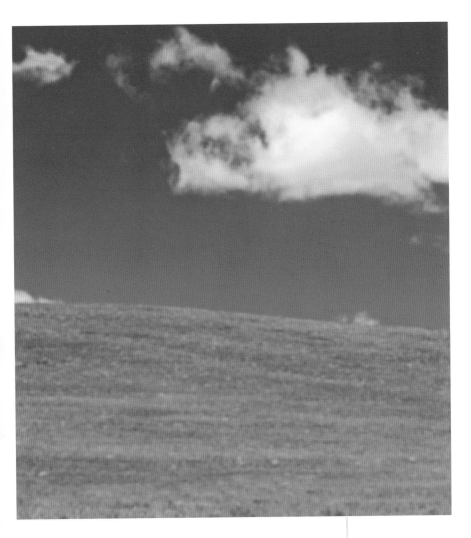

The Rules of Visualization

To visualize effectively, remember that the human framework has developed very specifically. When sitting, we balance on the spine and the muscles need to be harmonized. The spine, too, is important for the working of the nervous system. It is not possible to visualize effectively if you slouch or if the trunk is distorted.

171

Right Sit up straight against a wall or the back of an upright chair as you begin the process of visualization. Concentrate on your breathing. Close your eyes if you prefer to.

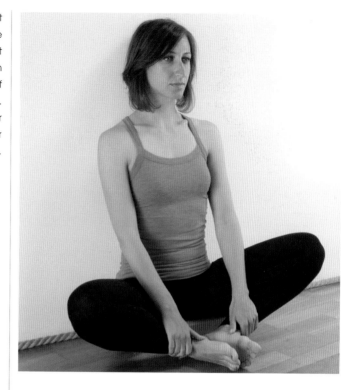

1 Unless you can already sit comfortably and correctly on the floor, use a chair or block. Close your eyes, and allow the head to balance comfortably on the shoulders. Wriggle the shoulders a little to ease any tension. Bring the hands together on the lap or place them on your ankles. Listen to the gentle sound of your breath: feel the cool touch of air on your nostrils as you breathe in and the warm flow of air as you breathe out. Feel the sense of relaxation as you breathe out.

2 Time is now irrelevant. The slow rhythm of your breath is like the comforting tick of a grandfather clock—it enhances the stillness, rather than detracts from it. When you are truly at ease, gently begin to bring in the visualization you have decided upon. Establish the feeling of it; let it flow all around you. This is to become your reality: you have gone into your own world and are now living fully in it.

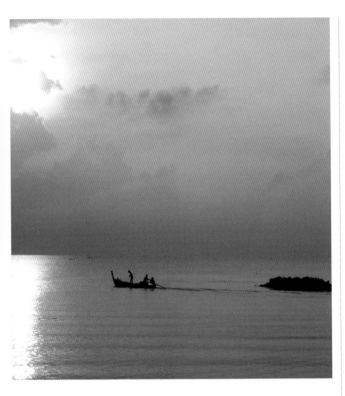

A Simple Visualization

Each breath we take is an intake of energy—not just from the flow of oxygen through the lungs, but by the stimulation of the body's electromagnetic force. In yoga, this is known as prana. It flows through the nervous system, stimulates the constant reinforcement of bone tissue, controls the heartbeat, and passes messages through the brain. Every cell in the body has its own electrical field, while the diaphragm acts as the pump of the whole system.

Sitting quietly, having checked your posture, concentrate on your breathing, making it· slow, rhythmic, and peaceful. Visualize your breath as you draw it in through your nostrils as a warm, soothing mist spreading as a warming flow up to the top of the head. Breathing slowly out, feel the breath flow through every part of your body, down to the tips of the toes. If any other thought intrudes, quietly

173

push it away and let this picture become totally real to you. Whatever happens, once the picture has formed in your mind, be sure not to let it leave you.

Continue for a minimum of five minutes (in due course, anything up to 20 minutes, or in fact, as long as you feel comfortable with). As you finish, let the visualization fade away, retaining the feeling of warming energy. Open your eyes and stretch.

Choosing an Image

In the early stages of visualization you can get into the right mood by recalling a time when everything felt good. A vacation perhaps, where the sense of peace and the warmth of the sun united to make you feel totally in harmony. Such recollections can help you create your own images.

Visualization in the Postures

The asanas largely developed from meditative practices. If you hold or use the body in a balanced position and then let your mind dwell on some beneficial concept, the body will naturally adapt itself, becoming more free and supple. This is not easy to achieve, but it brings great benefits. It is one of the unique aspects of yoga, setting it apart from other approaches.

Regular practice of the postures will ensure that they are performed with the minimum tension and with no waste of energy. As this happens, the visualization aspect can be introduced. Some of the postures you have been practicing should now be coming along well. When you are holding those that feel comfortable and balanced, let your mind dwell on a beautiful sunrise and experience that wonderful sensation of wellbeing it evokes. You will find that you can hold the posture better and it will be comfortable for longer.

Below If you are comfortable in some of the basic postures outlined in this book, why not try combining one or two of them with some positive visualization?

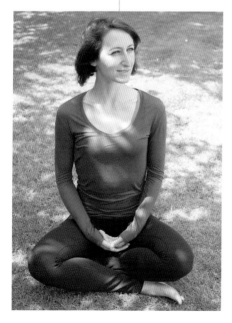

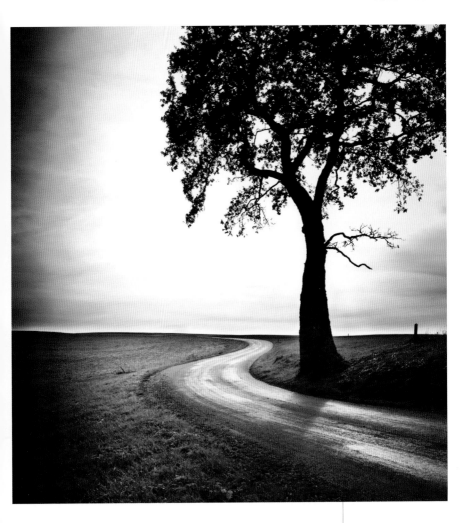

Set Your Own Guidelines

Always work with ideas that you find comfortable. For most people a beautiful dawn is inspiring, but a few may have had an unhappy experience that it could awaken. If so, choose another image. Remember, making progress in yoga is a two-way process. Absorb what you are taught, but never forget that you have your own role to play. When it comes to visualization, you are completely in charge.

Above Visualize whatever works for you—just ensure it is a peaceful scene.

175

Meditation

The four complementary aspects of human life are activation, relaxation, visualization, and meditation. All are essential to a truly fulfilled existence; all are the basic weapons of health and happiness.

Opposite There are many different ways in which to meditate, but the classic pose is illustrated here. Once again, the key factors for success are peace and quiet, as well as lack of clutter.

You are now using your body in association with the mind and the energy through the breath. You are stimulating your life through relaxation and visualization. Incorporating the peace of meditation is the next major step. As you progress, you will practice more asanas, but, even more importantly, deepen the way in which you use your body—not only when practicing yoga, but also in all aspects of life.

First Steps

What are the differences between relaxation, visualization, and meditation? In relaxation you allow the body to run, like an idling engine, while you observe but do not interfere. In visualization you use imagery to stimulate the functioning of the body. In meditation you withdraw the mind from the body (without losing awareness of its presence) and dwell on a single, non-physical concept. This takes you beyond the normal limitations of living, to achieve a much greater sense of control.

You can meditate sitting either in a chair or on the floor. It is not practical to meditate lying down. The conditions already explained (see page 172) apply here: the trunk must be comfortably upright, the hands together (or in a more classical position, in which thumb and forefinger of each hand are touching) and the eyes closed. Some schools of yoga advocate meditation with the eyes half-open, but most people find this extremely difficult. It is essential that the body should be comfortable, otherwise messages of distress are signaled to the brain and the calm mental basis is impossible.

There are countless ways of meditating and it is sensible to try several to find one that really suits you, but do not flutter about like a butterfly; that will not be helpful.

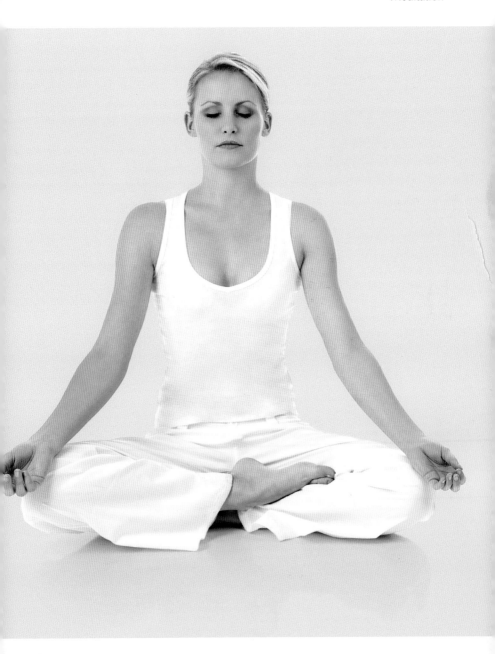

Hamsa Meditation

An image that has been used for centuries in Indian meditation is that of the wild goose or swan. These creatures are equally at home on land, water, or in the air. As such, they have come to symbolize the free spirit. An effective way to begin meditating is to sit correctly in a room where you will not be disturbed. Close your eyes and bring your mind to the flow and sound of your breath. After a minute or two visualize a goose or swan flying through the air. The Sanskrit word for the bird is Hamsa. Keep the visualization for a few minutes and then, as you breathe in, repeat to yourself, "Ham," as you breathe out, repeat, "sa." "Ham ... sa."

Now let the vision of the bird fade, but continue to repeat, "Ham ... sa" together with the in- and out-breath. Any stray thoughts which intrude should be gently pushed away and the chanting resumed. Initially, around ten minutes is long enough. Gradually you can extend this and, before long, between 20 and 30 minutes will become ideal.

As you get more used to the practice, you will not only find that your mind is both peaceful and alert, but your body will also feel lithe and supple, for the physical benefits of meditation are considerable.

Below The image of geese flying across a peaceful sky has been a mainstay of Indian meditation for many hundreds of years.

Top Tips for Successful Yoga Meditation

• **Choose a convenient time**
Meditation is essentially relaxation time, so it should be done entirely at your own convenience. So, for all meditations, choose a time when you know you are not likely to be disturbed and are free to relax and enjoy the experience. The hours of sunrise and sunset, while nature switches between day and night, are also ideal for the practice.

• **Choose a quiet place**
Just like a convenient hour, choose a place where you are not likely to be disturbed. Quiet and peaceful surroundings will make the meditation experience more enjoyable and relaxing.

• **Sit comfortably**
Your posture makes a difference, too. Make sure you are relaxed, comfortable, and steady. Sit straight with your spine erect; keep your shoulders and neck relaxed, and eyes closed throughout the process. You do not have to sit in Padmasana (the lotus position) to meditate if you find it difficult or uncomfortable.

• **Keep a relatively empty stomach**
A good time to meditate is before having a meal. After eating, there is a danger that you might doze off while meditating. However, do not force yourself to meditate when you are very hungry.

• **Begin with a few warm-up exercises**
A few warm-up or sukshma yoga exercises before sitting to meditate help improve circulation, removes inertia and restlessness, and makes the body feel lighter. You will be able to sit steadily for a longer time.

• **Take a few deep breaths**
This is again preparation for easy meditation. Deep breathing in and out before meditating is always a good idea. This helps to steady the rhythm of the breath and leads the mind into a peaceful meditative state.

Breathing During Meditation

Pranayama, the yogic art of breath control, was introduced in the section on breathing for yoga on pages 30–31. Once you have mastered the basics of breath control, you can begin to experiment with different postures while practicing it, as well as exploring the yogic art of lengthening the breath.

Which Postures Are Suitable?

Eventually, you can perform breathing exercises sitting in an upright posture, such as the Lotus (see pages 154–55), the Hero (see pages 72–3), the Tailor (see pages 80–81), or Easy Cross-Legged pose (see pages 78–9). The posture must be done well, so that the body is evenly balanced and the spine remains lifted throughout. Refining and maintaining a good sitting posture for Pranayama needs to be learned in person from a teacher, so perform the technique given here lying down.

Lengthening the Breath

Lie down, with your eyes closed, in the Supported Corpse pose (see page 135) and rest for a few minutes, observing your breathing as it takes place naturally. When your body is quiet and the rhythm of your breathing has settled, practice extending first the inhalation and then the exhalation through the following exercises. As you breathe, use your lungs evenly and keep your breath flowing smoothly. Breathe through your nose.

1 Normal in-breath; slow, controlled out-breath. First, breathe out more fully than usual but without effort. Inhale normally. Exhale steadily and slowly, so the out-breath lasts longer than usual. Do not strain or make the breath noisy. Then inhale normally again. Exhale slowly and deeply. Continue with this pattern for about five minutes, without strain. After a slow exhalation, return to normal breathing and relax.

2 Normal out-breath; slow, controlled in-breath. After a full out-breath, inhale steadily and slowly, keeping the breath smooth and evenly filling both lungs. Do not inflate your abdomen, but let

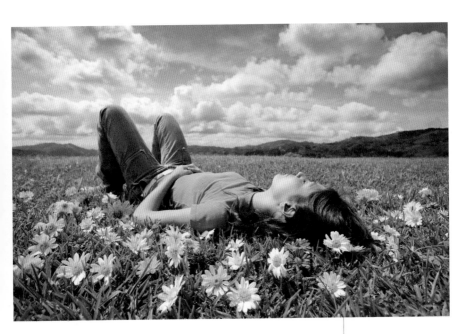

your ribcage expand upward, forward, and sideways. Breathe out normally. Again, inhale in a slow, controlled way, without tension or strain. Breathe out normally. Continue with this pattern for about five minutes. After this, you should relax for a while. This may be enough to begin with. When you are comfortable with this preliminary practice, continue to the next stage.

3 Slow, controlled in-breath and out-breath. After lying, relaxing, and observing your breathing, exhale completely. Breathe in steadily and slowly, as before. Then exhale, also steadily and slowly. Continue this pattern of long, slow inhalations and exhalations, without tension or strain. After about five minutes, finish on a slow exhalation, then breathe normally and rest. Gently turn onto your side, so you can move the support from under your back. Lie down flat, with a folded blanket under your head. Relax in the Corpse position (see pages 129–31) for a few minutes. Finish by opening your eyes, bending your knees, and turning onto your right side for a while. Then roll on to your left side, rest there for a while, and get up.

Above Visualize your breath entering and leaving your body and relax completely.

181

Sitting in Meditation

When concentration is uninterrupted and the mind is totally absorbed in the object of contemplation, meditation takes place. The mind is undisturbed by sensory concerns yet fully aware and alive. This is hard to achieve and cannot be forced. A skillful teacher can give encouragement, advice, and explanation. Ultimately, meditation can be experienced in any posture; it need not be confined to a particular time of day, place, or activity. However, a balanced posture, in which the spine is upright and the body relaxed yet alert, favors the mental conditions that allow meditation to occur. The Easy Cross-Legged position (see pages 78–9) can be a good choice, or the Perfect Pose (Siddhasana), which is described here.

The Perfect Pose: Siddhasana

1 Sit on a folded blanket or similar support if your hips are stiff or your lower back tips back. Bend your left leg and bring the foot in towards the center line of the body, placing the top of the foot on the floor and the heel in front of the pubis.

2 Fold your right leg similarly and bring your right heel over the left. Tuck the right toes in between your left calf and thigh. The knees are wide apart, the high points of the heels in line with the center of your body, and your spine erect.

3 Stretch your arms and rest the back of your hands on your knees. You can join the tip of your index finger to that of the thumb, keeping the other fingers extended. This is Jnana mudra: the symbol of knowledge.

4 When practicing this with the other postures, repeat, folding your legs the other way. If using Siddhasana for meditation or breathing, it is not necessary to change the cross of your legs during the session. Instead, close your eyes and look within, focusing your attention and stilling your mind.

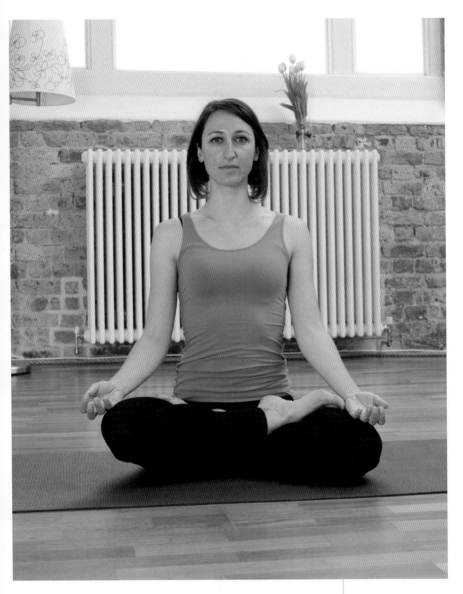

Candle Meditation

The first requirement of meditation is the power to concentrate—darana in Sanskrit. The realization of this helps you to understand how important meditation is, for everyone knows the value of concentration. The object is to direct the mind to dwell exclusively on one subject. At school, children are urged to concentrate and from then on people realize how important concentration is in order to achieve their goals. Yet, in everyday life, we are seldom taught how to concentrate. Meditation, therefore, offering techniques of concentration, is a valuable aid to all aspects of life, from carrying out mundane daily activities to finding a deep peace of mind.

Meditating on a lit candle is a very old practice. It is gentle and calming. It is also a comparatively easy introduction to the art of concentration. Sit erect on the floor or in a chair, having placed the candle a short distance in front of you where you can see it clearly. Gaze steadily at the candle flame for two or three minutes, noting first of all its outline—how steady it is, how it flickers—and then the colors in the flame. Now cover your eyes with your palms and continue to gaze on the image of the candle, which will remain. Continue to note movement and color. As the mind's image of the flame begins

Right Meditation with the help of a candle is another centuries-old practice of yoga that is designed to calm and still the mind.

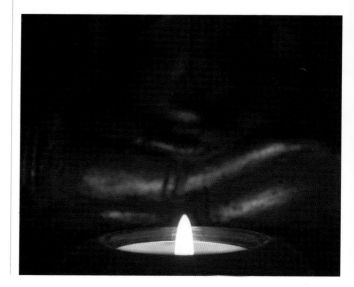

to fade, remove the hands from the eyes, keeping them closed, and maintain awareness of the flame even though you can no longer see it. As and when this awareness fades, gently open your eyes. With practice, the final period of awareness will become longer and longer. It can only be maintained through concentration.

Using Sound

The combination of sound and vision can provide a deep basis for concentration, as we have already seen through the "Hamsa" meditation (see page 178). It has been an Eastern concept for thousands of years that the sound of "Om" (Au-uu-m) is the most sacred of all sounds. It is still chanted daily and, it is claimed, this was the basis of the chant "Amen," used at the end of prayers, hymns, and psalms in Christian services.

In the 17th century, the astronomer Johannes Kepler declared that each planet had a "song" and he wrote down the individual notations. A few years ago, a professor of music and a professor of geology in the United States took Kepler's laws and notations and applied them to the motions of the planets. This was fed into a computer connected to a music synthesizer. The result was a "song" of the planets—just as Kepler had argued! If planets in motion must project sound, clearly the sum total of all the objects in motion throughout the universe will also provide a sound. One day we may be able to record this, and no doubt, it will be found to be "Om"— the sound of the universe.

Again, sitting correctly, with the eyes closed, first pay attention to the calm and peaceful rhythm of your breath. After a minute or two, repeat the sound Om (Au-uu-m) to yourself each time you breathe out. Get swept up in the sound, filling your mind, your body, the room … everything with it. If your concentration slips, pay attention to your breath and, after a minute or two, open your eyes.

Practice Makes Perfect

As with other forms of practice, the more often you perform this, the longer the periods of total concentration you can achieve. You will find the vibration of this amazing sound brings a feeling of harmony that stays with you.

Feeling the Energy Flow

There is no time when mind and body are not working together, with the brain acting as the go-between. Nobody knows the degree to which we create our own reality, but there are, for example, authenticated cases of stigmata—people actually producing bleeding wounds on their hands and feet by identifying totally in the mind with the Crucifixion. We know that the link between mind and body can be harmful, but we often fail to realize that a strong positive mind/body link can be as beneficial as a negative one can be harmful. Einstein demonstrated that matter equals energy; without energy there is no existence. Energy is a flow—there may be whirls, eddies, torrents, quiet little trickles, but in every aspect it must flow. To be out of ease means a lack of or obstruction to the flow of energy: literally, dis-ease.

The section on visualization has already outlined the process of creating an effective flow of energy. Carefully monitored tests have shown practitioners changing their body temperature (sometimes in specifically chosen parts of the body), reducing their blood pressure and even controlling the beat of the heart. With practice, we can all change aspects of our functioning for the better.

Use the visualization of the flow of energy to tone your whole being, enhancing body function and stimulating mental activity. The sitting position is ideal, either on the floor or in a chair. Keep the back erect but not stiff; link the hands.

Golden Mist

With the eyes closed, allow yourself to pay attention to the breath: it should be quite slow and above all rhythmic. Become aware of the in-breath by feeling the cool flow of the air on the nostrils. Create the impression that the air is a golden mist, sun-like in nature. As you breathe in, this golden mist links with the warmth of your body and rises to the top of your head. As you breathe out, it flows right down through every part of the body into the fingers and toes.

The object of this process is, through calm persistence, to identify more and more with this warm, golden flow; to be a part of its rise and fall; to feel it move into every nook and cranny of the body. Your whole being becomes one harmonious rhythm: a glorious ballet movement, a wave of silk in the breeze, an undulation of water in the ocean.

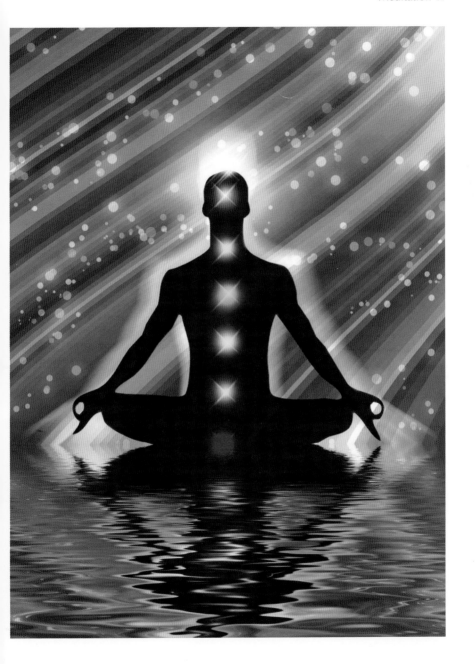

Instant Relaxation

It is so easy to let things cause you stress that you tend to think it is inevitable, and that you can do nothing about it. Many major problems start with minor ones that go uncorrected and just grow, almost undetected.

Right at the start of this book, the need for stretching, releasing the neck and shoulders, and simply swinging energy into the body were emphasized. All these quite simple things need to become a part of life, used when the body signals tension or lack of energy.

Other equally simple actions are shown here in a yoga studio setting, but they could be performed equally well in the home or elsewhere.

1 Many activities cramp the body, slow circulation, and limit muscle function. To counteract this, work the shoulders and the back for a minute or so, then take the hands and link the fingers as you place them on the back of the head, elbows out.

2 Take a deep breath in and, as you breathe out, press the head down, bringing the chin against the neck and the elbows closer together. Feel the strong stretch on the back of the neck. Hold the position until you feel the need to breathe in again and then release. Repeat at least three times.

Much of our time at work is spent with back and shoulders hunched, due to sitting at desks in front of computers and other machines all day long. This is uncomfortable in the short term and can become serious in time. Apart from the sitting stretch, also perform the standing one already shown (see pages 32–3), even if it is not practical to carry out the whole sequence.

It is not always practical to get up and move about; an effective stretch can be carried out while seated in a chair. Link the fingers,

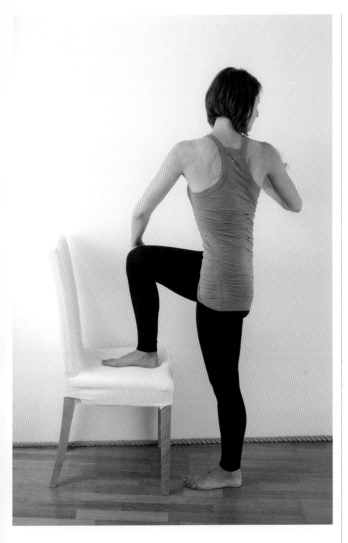

Left You can perform any number of beneficial and muscle-relaxing stretches with the aid of a chair—either sitting or standing.

letting hands lie on the lap. Breathe in, stretch the arms into the air, turning the hands so that the palms are uppermost. Get the arms level with the ears and straighten them, still stretching up. Hold until the impulse comes to breathe out and then come slowly down. This also should be repeated at least three times.

189

Upside Down Again

Is it natural to upend ourselves? You have only to look at children playing to get the answer—they love cartwheels, handstands, and rolling over and over.

Keeping the body active and even turning it upside down is a naturally inherited instinct. The inverted positions of yoga rationalize this instinct, to our mental and physical benefit. The Plough is a topsy-turvy posture that is physically stimulating and mentally calming. While yoga asanas are performed with control, the swing and sense of balance we all had as uninhibited children are essential for effective performance. This posture can also be performed with support.

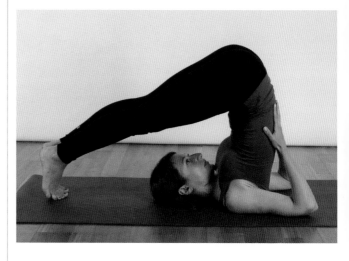

The Plough

1 Lie on the floor, feet together, arms by the sides, palms down. Breathe quite deeply and, on an in-breath, swing the legs into the air, using arms and hands to provide both pressure and balance.

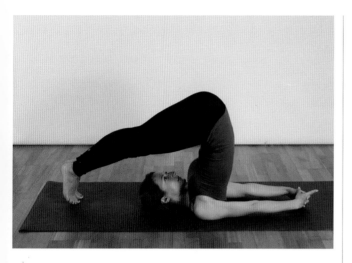

2 When you feel balanced on the shoulders, bring up the arms and hold ankles or shins. The arms are straight, not bent at the elbows. Retain the position, preferably with the eyes closed, breathing gently. Gradually develop a floating feeling. Hold it for as long as is comfortable. Bring the arms back to the floor first to control the slow lowering of the legs.

3 Remove the hands from the legs, lowering the legs until the toes touch the floor. Maintain balance by letting the fingers lightly support the back. When coming down, bring the arms to the floor first and use them to control the slow movement of the legs. Relax for a minute or two.

Regaining Childish Zest
Getting back childish zest is an important aspect of adult practice: you need to combine that instinct with thoughtfulness. While the slow, controlled performance is central to yoga, you can often make progress by first of all coming back to the roll-about aspect of childhood and, from this, impose the greater control learned as an adult.

Controlling Our Responses

Life is a series of challenges and how people meet these over the years will play a major role in their outlook and health. It has been shown that happy events can challenge people as much as unhappy ones; all are aspects of that much-used word: stress.

Opposite Sometimes, the best reaction to stress is simply to remind yourself that you are alive and that the world is a wonderful place. Leaping into the air can often help, too!

No one can avoid stressful events, but it is possible to control reactions to them. Classically, yoga texts urge that both happy and unhappy events be treated with dispassion. Few will achieve this, but it is not difficult to bring about beneficial modifications.

Bad news affects breathing, which in turn tenses the muscles of the trunk. The flow of energy to the brain, too, is impaired, making clear thinking difficult. If something bad happens, sit quietly, place the hands on the chest, deliberately slow your breathing, and be aware of your control both of breathing in and breathing out. In a minute or two you will feel the pressure ease.

Even good news can upset your equilibrium. To accept good news calmly and effectively, bring the hands, palms downward at chest level, and feel you are pushing down the gasping sensation which arises. Let the hands rise a little as you breathe in and descend slowly on the out-breath. Again, ensure that the breath is slowed.

Changing

Reactions to life events become firm reflexes and are hard to change. But change is possible and where these reactions are damaging—which is all too often the case—it is important to work to bring it about. For example, the rushing person, always looking at his or her watch and dashing from one thing to the next, can be helped by simply sticking a little colored circle on the watch-face. Every time the watch is looked at there is a reminder of the need to slow down. Encourage the breathing to slow and the annoyance will abate.

192

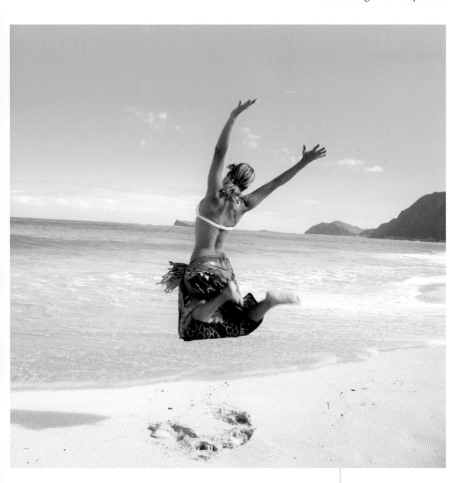

If something causes worry, you tend to feel that your head is spinning and that you can't quite grasp what is going on. As with all these emotions, conscious slowing and quieting of the breath is essential and, in this case, placing the fingertips gently on the forehead helps to reduce the mental turmoil.

Irritating or annoying news can, if not checked, lead to harmful reactions. Bringing the hands on to the chest in the prayer position (namaste) has a calming effect, just by its body language. If all else fails, doing something physical can also often have a beneficial effect.

193

Uniting Body and Mind

Using the body to quiet the mind and enhance inner peace, together with the capacity to act, is a concept little understood in the West. Using the body is considered to be a physical process only and using the mind is not really understood at all.

I f these two central aspects of life are brought together, your whole outlook changes. You come to realize there is a new dimension to living. The examples given in this book are only "for instances." The one below will probably be something of a surprise, because it is a variation on a standard form of stretching.

1 Standing with the legs just a little apart, breathe out and as you breathe in stretch the arms out to the side and over the head. Lift high.

2 Then, start stretching up with the right arm, pulling up the· whole of the right side.

3 Alternate with the left arm and, after at least a dozen times with each arm, have a final strong stretch up with both arms. Bring the arms down on an out-breath. While performing the stretch fill yourself with a feeling of rejoicing. Liberate your body.

The Simple Tree

Mental and physical balance go together, something which is not fully realized. Prayer in India is often combined with physical movements. Today you still see devotees standing on the banks of the Ganges, balanced on one leg, with the hands in the namaste (prayer position) on the chest. Their eyes are closed and they are reciting a prayer.

1 Place one foot on the opposite knee, letting the knee of the bent leg fall outward. Place the hands together on the chest and close

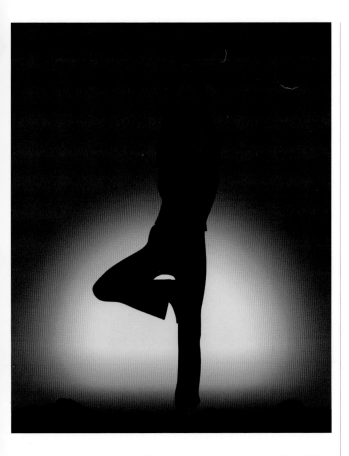

the eyes. Repeat to yourself a thought or saying you find helpful, or say a prayer. The length of time you can hold this will increase with practice. Repeat the process with the other leg.

Teaching Yourself

Yoga is a process of self-realization. While this book aims to provide information and hints on how to proceed, you, the reader, are your own most valuable teacher. Any book can do no more than provide a few examples, for the subject is immense. Once you have grasped the concept that the body functions better when a calm, controlled mind lets it do so, you can then apply the idea to a whole variety of postures.

195

Energy and the Chakras

The human body is a mass of electromagnetic fields, in an electro-magnetic world, which is part of an electromagnetic universe. Keeping all this in balance are the mystical "chakras."

Below Ancient oriental cultures have believed in the chakras—internal energy forces in the human body that link inextricably with those of nature—for many centuries.

S ome of the body's electric energy is generated by the pumping of the heart, but "no man is an island" and we share this wonderful mixture of waves, vibrations, electromagnetism, and gases, which is termed the air or the atmosphere. The term used for it in yoga is prana, which can be translated as "lifeforce."

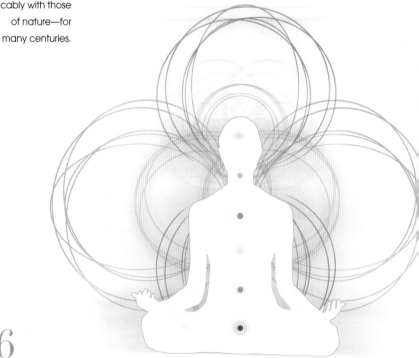

196

Energy Centers

Electromagnetically based energy flows through the body and corresponds with the Chinese concept of acupuncture, now recognized in the West and used by many doctors. The yoga concept is that the body has a series of energy centers, known as chakras. (Chakra means a wheel or vortex.) These are situated parallel with the spine. While yet insufficiently researched, the evidence for the existence of these centers is growing.

SAHASRARA CHAKRA provides the link between the individual and the universal.

AJNA CHAKRA, the chakra of command, links with the hypothalamus and pituitary glands, which order much of our mind-body reactions.

VISHUDDA CHAKRA, in the area of the laryngeal plexus, is concerned with steadiness and balance.

ANAHATA CHAKRA, at the heart center (cardiac plexus), links with emotions over living things ("made my heart flutter").

MANIPURA CHAKRA, at the point of the solar plexus (technically the coeliac plexus), is associated with gastric fire ("fire in the belly") and emotions concerning "inanimate" aspects of life, such as examinations.

SVADISHTHANA CHAKRA is concerned with water, sexual flow, and the sense of taste.

MULADHARA CHAKRA, in the groin area, is related to excretion and the sense of smell.

Creating Balance

For thousands of years, yoga teachings have insisted that human beings have one aspect of energy or force on one side of the body and a different one on the other, the two interlinking to provide a balanced life.

Opposite Good balance is both the key to yoga and a happy life. It is important to remember that this balance should be as much mental as it is physical.

The force on the left side, called Ida, is related to the coolness of the moon and is the calculating aspect of life. That on the right, Pingala, relates to the warmth of the sun and the process of creativity.

In recent years, neuroscientists have established that the left hemisphere of the brain is associated with verbal activity and numeracy—the cool, calculating aspects—and the right hemisphere controls our creative processes—in other words, exactly what the yogis had been saying for centuries.

The importance of balance in life is a question of balance. Tension, or willpower, is necessary but it must be balanced with relaxation, or letting go. This "letting go" is based upon the in-and-out flow of the breath, upon which all mental and physical functions are based.

Self-awareness, the basis of consciousness, is an instrument by which life can be both developed and enhanced mentally and physically. If, however, you abrogate control of the brain, you abrogate control of life itself; used negatively, self-awareness can become destructive. The choice between creation or destruction lies in our own hands.

Once you are aware, you can use that awareness either positively or negatively. The brain and the body are actually the servants of consciousness.

Bearing in mind the need for balance in all things—sometimes called the middle way—you can review your life and see how far you make use of the cool, logical aspects on the one hand and how far you indulge in creativity in all its forms on the other. The brain is divided into two hemispheres: the left hemisphere controls the calculating aspects of life, the right controls creativity.

198

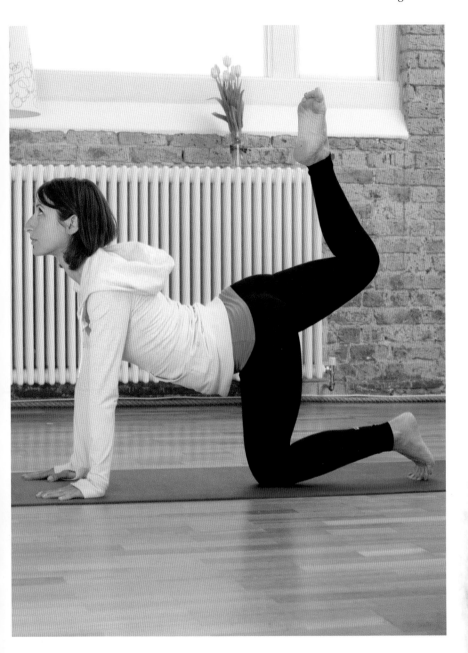

Countering the Senses

The messages our senses provide are thought of as "reality." In fact, sensory reaction is determined by circumstances and habit. Yoga has the power to change these instinctive reactions.

Below Even if it is stiflingly hot, yoga can train your mind to counter your senses and believe the opposite. This can be useful in controlling pain and living a more settled life, amongst many other advantages.

For example, in a temperate country, where the temperature was 68°F (20°C), a native inhabitant would regard it as a nice, warm day, a visitor newly arrived from Alaska would find it stiflingly hot, while another from Central Africa would be shivering in the cold. Similar analogies can be provided for the other senses. However, it is important to realize that the senses are very useful but no one should be a slave to them —and yoga can be incredibly helpful in this teaching.

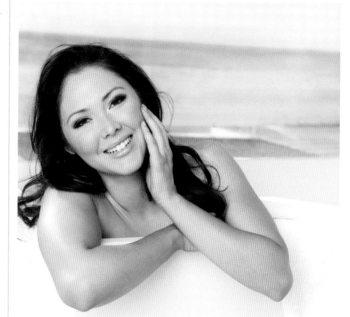

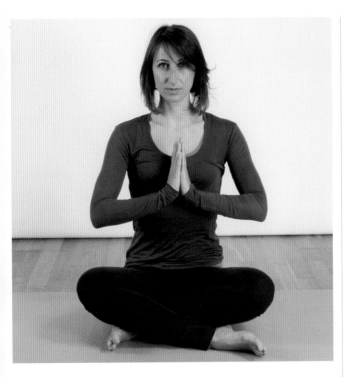

One effective way of countering a feeling of coolness or cold is to sit correctly, with the eyes closed and recollect a vacation in which you lay on a beach in hot sunshine. If some feeling of cold persists, recall that coming out of the water you have felt a little chilly until the sun has dried your body and again you feel the sun at work. If you do this calmly and with assurance, you will be surprised at the result. You can use the same technique, with a corresponding visualization, to counteract feeling overheated. In both cases, the strength of your concentration will make the brain respond to the visualization, rather than the senses.

The yoga philosophy develops a spirit of detachment in which the signals of the senses are regarded as useful indicators, but not necessarily as imperative demands. The resulting mental stability, when such a state is achieved, establishes a brain/body harmony that makes for balance, conservation of energy, and enhanced well-being.

201

The Yoga Day

Yoga offers a singularly comprehensive approach to life: profound thoughts about existence and the universe on one hand, and how to avoid the pitfalls that generate both unhappiness and illness on the other.

As you know, water dripping constantly can make a hole in a stone. Our inability to react effectively to small challenges creates a mental and physical build-up which can be very damaging. Try to counteract this by planning your days more effectively.

Early Morning

Remember the importance of opening up the breath, de-tensing, and stretching. Setting a standard for the day with a thought or a short reading can be of immense benefit. Build up concentration, too, by doing chores, such as washing, cleaning your teeth, brushing your hair, with care. Doing one thing and thinking of another leads to confusion.

Mid-Morning

Remember that you can concentrate for relatively short periods —effectively for about an hour. Take regular short breaks. A few minutes' relief will actually heighten your capacity to understand and remember. Saying, "I'm too busy to stop" will usually end in slipshod results. All too often over-concentration and physical tension go together. Even small movements like working the shoulders and the neck can make a big difference. Above all, pay attention to the need for quiet, natural breathing.

Lunchtime

Digestion is a complex process. Snatching a snack can be harmful and slouching over a meal can turn the digestive process into a torture. Getting into the habit of eating carefully will pay dividends.

Afternoon

The afternoon can be quite a dangerous time! Digestion is a slow process, requiring an effective flow of blood in the abdominal area. Good erect posture will help health and happiness by allowing the system to function well. Mental and physical capacity is generally lowered for a while. A short rest, a walk, or some other sensible way of letting the body function quietly can be immensely beneficial. Millions of people these days work in front of computers and other apparatus, and all these things tend to affect posture, diminish energy levels, and interfere with the effective working of the muscles. Good posture, calm breathing, and regular short breaks are essential.

Early Evening

For very many people, the early evening is a transition period, moving from work into evening activities. This is one of the best times to combine a wash, bath, or shower with at least a short session of yoga asanas, followed by relaxation and awareness of breathing. With such a break, one feels a "new person." Energy is topped up and the evening becomes far more enjoyable.

Bedtime

Too many people allow the day to build up mental and physical tensions, and then jump straight into bed, only to wonder why they do not sleep properly. Preparing for bed requires getting the mind into a relaxed state, so that sleep can follow naturally. Some gentle, but effective, stretching helps to start this process, and a few minutes of calm, rhythmic breathing will underline the process. It is good, also, to remind oneself that the capacity to deal with matters on the following day will depend, at least in part, on a good night's sleep. In bed, listen to the breath, and liken it to the wavelets of a calm sea breaking on the shore.

Many people may feel that such simple, everyday matters cannot be linked with yoga, but an examination of the traditional writings reveals that yogis have always understood that the small points of life are closely linked to the big issues. If we establish a simple but effective pattern to see us through each day, then the major activities and challenges will be dealt with much more effectively.

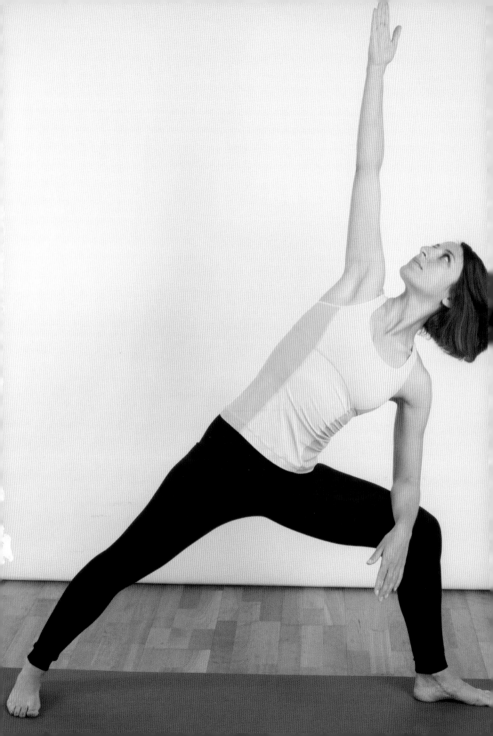

Daily Routines

Daily yoga practice is beneficial, but these routines are helpful even if you practice less frequently. The practice sessions are given in four sets of three. The postures are listed in the order in which they should be practiced. Start with the first three sessions, alternating them until you feel ready to learn more postures. Then work on the next three routines, and so on. At first, you will probably need to refer back frequently to the pages in the main text that describe how each posture is done. The more difficult postures are not included in the session plans; a yoga class will help you incorporate these into your practice sessions when you are ready.

Beginning Postures

During your first sessions, the main challenge is learning how to work in the basic standing poses. Aim to grasp the overall shape of each pose you attempt. Do not be over ambitious.

Recognize your current limitations and use supports to help you, where recommended. As you progress through these sessions, you will start to develop the sense of where your body is in space and how your weight is distributed. Enjoy each new opportunity to stretch your legs, arms, and spine.

Watch Points
- You do not need to master every posture completely before trying something new, but do not rush on too quickly; progress comes with enthusiasm, persistence, sensitivity, and patience.
- Do not remain in the postures for a long time at first; it is better to repeat them. As you become stronger, you may find that you can hold them longer.
- Where postures are repeated on one side and then the other, do each side for the same amount of time.
- Use supports sensibly.
- Pay attention to cautions, and practice only postures appropriate to your condition (see Introduction, pages 8–27).

Session 1

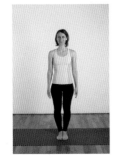

1 Mountain (p. 44)

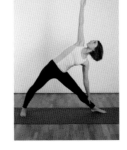

2 Triangle (p. 52)

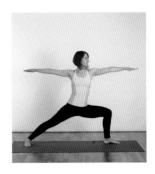

3 Warrior II (p. 58)

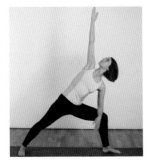

4 Horizon (p. 54)

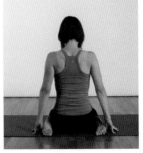

5 Hero (p. 72)

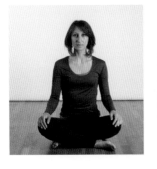

6 Easy Cross-Legged (p. 78)

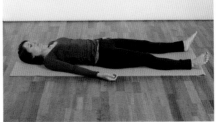

7 Corpse (p. 129)

Session 2

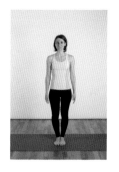

1 Mountain (p. 44)

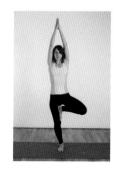

2 Tree (p. 48)

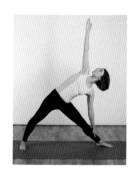

3 Triangle (p. 18)

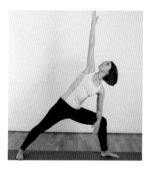

4 Horizon (p. 54)

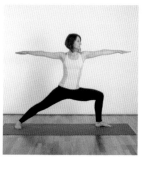

5 Warrior II (p. 58)

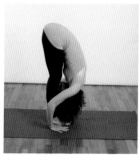

6 Standing Forward Bend (p. 62)

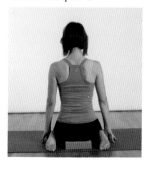

7 Hero (p. 72)

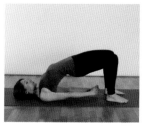

8 Bridge (p. 112)

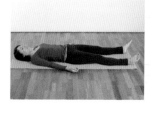

9 Corpse (p. 129)

Session 3

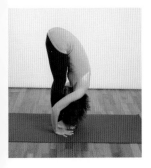 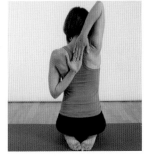 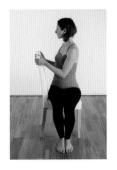

1 Standing Forward Bend (p. 62) **2** Cow's Head (p. 74)   **3** Bharadvajasana I (p. 94)

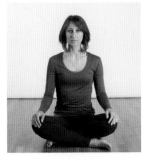 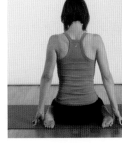

4 Easy Cross-Legged (p. 78)   **5** Hero (p. 72)

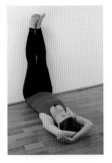 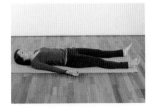

6 Legs up Against a Wall (p. 110)   **7** Corpse (p. 129)

Extending Your Skills

In these sessions, more forward stretching is added, so you can concentrate on learning to straighten your legs fully.

D raw up your front thigh muscles to support the knee joints and release tension on the backs of your legs. Check the alignment of your straight legs; the knee should face the same way as the toes of that leg, and the feet should be positioned as directed for the posture. The Shoulder Stand (Sarvangasana), in various forms, is introduced. It is a key posture, and it is important to understand how to work in it safely.

Watch Points
- You do not need to master every posture completely before trying something new, but do not rush on too quickly; progress comes with enthusiasm, persistence, sensitivity, and patience.
- Do not remain in the postures for a long time at first; it is better to repeat them. As you become stronger, you may find that you can hold them longer.
- Where postures are repeated on one side and then the other, do each side for the same amount of time.
- Use supports sensibly.
- Pay attention to cautions, and practice only postures appropriate to your condition (see Introduction, pages 8–27).

Session 1

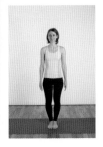

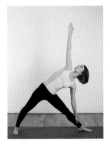

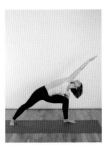

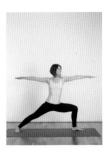

1 Mountain (p. 44)   **2** Triangle (p. 52)   **3** Horizon (p. 54)   **4** Warrior II (p. 58)

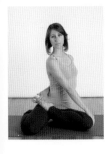

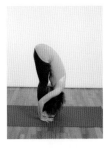

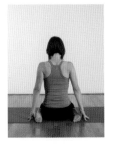

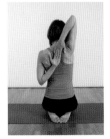

5 The Twist (p. 164)   **6** Standing Forward Bend (p. 62)   **7** Hero (p. 72)   **8** Cow's Head (p. 74)

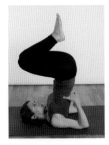

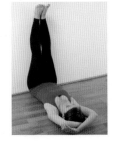

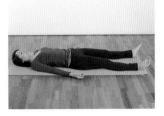

9 Starter Shoulder Stand (p. 118)   **10** Legs up against a Wall (p. 110)   **11** Corpse (p. 129)

Session 2

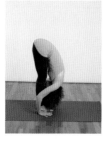

1 Standing Forward Bend (p. 62)

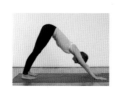

2 Dog (p. 64)

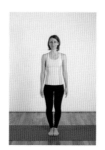

3 Mountain (p. 44)

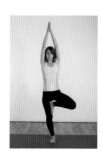

4 Tree (p. 48)

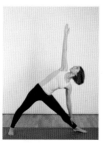

5 Triangle (p. 52)

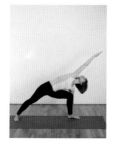

6 Horizon (p. 54)

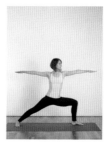

7 Warrior II (p. 58)

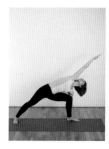

8 Horizon (p. 54)

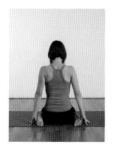

9 Hero (p. 72)

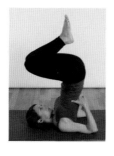

10 Starter Shoulder Stand (p. 118)

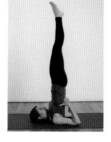

11 Shoulder Stand (p. 120)

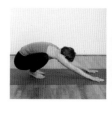

12 Garland (p. 88)

Session 3

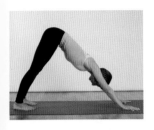

1 Dog (p. 64)

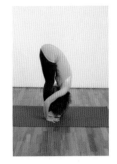

2 Standing Forward Bend (p. 62)

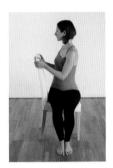

3 Bharadvajasana I (p. 94)

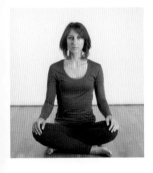

4 Easy Cross-Legged (p. 78)

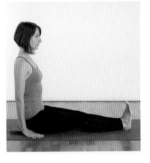

5 Staff (p. 68)

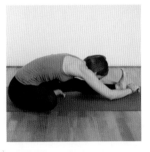

6 Head-to-Knee Bend (p. 84)

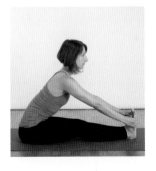

7 Seated Forward Bend (p. 70)

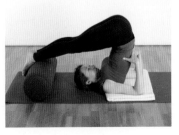

8 Supported Plough (p. 122)

213

Adding More Postures

By the time you reach this stage, you will be familiar with many of the postures. Improve your stability and understanding of the poses that you know and use your growing understanding to work in the new postures as you add them.

Y ou are likely to use supports for many of the positions included in this section; think carefully about how these can help you to do the pose more accurately and with less strain. Take your time as you assess the best way to go about these postures, taking into account your personal level of proficiency and experience in yoga.

Watch Points
- You do not need to master every posture completely before trying something new, but do not rush on too quickly; progress comes with enthusiasm, persistence, sensitivity, and patience.
- Do not remain in the postures for a long time at first; it is better to repeat them. As you become stronger, you may find that you can hold them longer.
- Where postures are repeated on one side and then the other, do each side for the same amount of time.
- Use supports sensibly.
- Pay attention to cautions, and practice only postures appropriate to your condition (see Introduction, pages 8–27).

Session 1

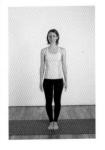

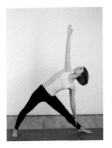

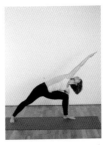

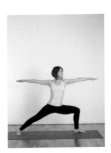

1 Mountain (p. 44)

2 Triangle (p. 52)

3 Horizon (p. 54)

4 Warrior II (p. 58)

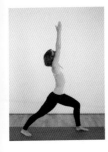

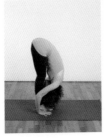

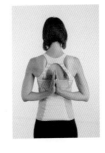

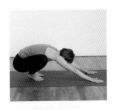

5 Warrior I (p. 56)

6 Standing Forward Bend (p. 62)

7 Reverse Prayer (p. 60)

8 The Garland (p. 88)

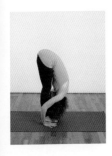

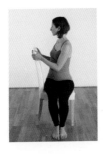

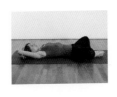

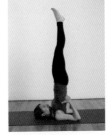

9 Forward Bend, Feet Wide (p. 62)

10 Bharadvajasana I (p. 94)

11 Reclining Tailor (p. 100)

12 Shoulder Stand (p. 120)

215

13 Plough (p. 122); 14 Corpse (p. 129) (not shown).

Session 2

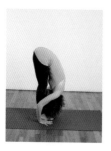 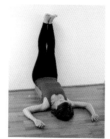 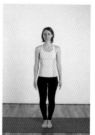 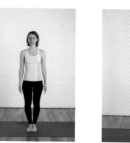

1 Standing Forward Bend (p. 62)

2 Leg Raising (p. 116)

3 Mountain (p. 44)

4 Tree (p. 48)

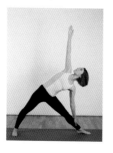 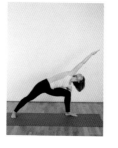 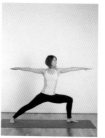 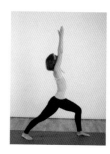

5 Triangle (p.52)

6 Horizon (p. 54)

7 Warrior II (p. 58)

8 Warrior I (p. 56)

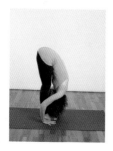 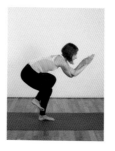 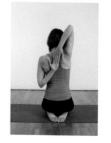 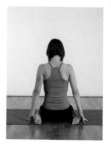

9 Standing Forward Bend (p. 62)

10 Eagle (p. 50)

11 Cow's Head (p. 74)

12 Hero (p. 72)

13 Shoulder Stand (p. 120); I4 Plough (p. 122); 15 Forward Bend (p. 70); 16 Corpse (p. 129) (not shown).

Session 3

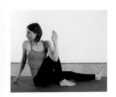

1 Maricy's pose III (p. 92)

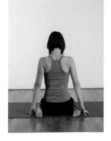

2 Hero (p. 72)

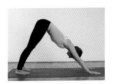

3 Dog (p. 64)

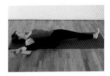

4 Leg Stretching (p. 108)

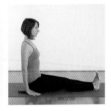

5 Staff (p. 68)

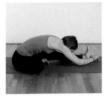

6 Head-to-Knee Bend (p. 84)

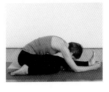

7 One-Leg-Forward Bend (p. 62)

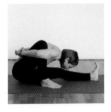

8 Maricy's Pose I (p. 90)

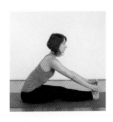

9 Seated Forward Bend (p. 70)

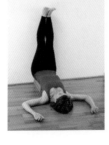

10 Raised Hips and Legs (p. 116)

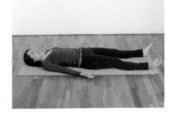

11 Corpse (p. 129)

Consolidation

These sessions are slightly longer and introduce the remaining basic postures. If you do not have enough time, follow one of the earlier sessions, or adapt these plans to fit your schedule.

As a general rule, begin your sessions with simple stretches that help you to focus on what you are doing and prepare your body for the more demanding postures. End each session with quiet poses and relaxation. Plan additional sessions in the light of the advice given by your teacher and what you learn from your own experience.

Watch Points
- You do not need to master every posture completely before trying something new, but do not rush on too quickly; progress comes with enthusiasm, persistence, sensitivity, and patience.
- Do not remain in the postures for a long time at first; it is better to repeat them. As you become stronger, you may find that you can hold them longer.
- Where postures are repeated on one side and then the other, do each side for the same amount of time.
- Use supports sensibly.
- Pay attention to cautions, and practice only postures appropriate to your condition (see Introduction, pages 8–27).

Session 1

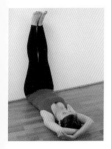

1 Leg Raising (p. 108)

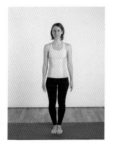

2 Mountain (p. 44)

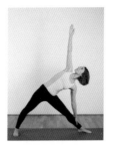

3 Triangle (p. 52)

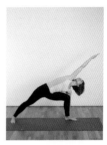

4 Horizon (p. 54)

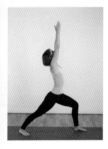

5 Warrior I (p. 22)

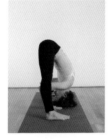

6 Standing Forward Bend (p. 62)

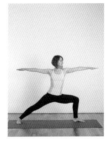

7 Warrior II (p. 58)

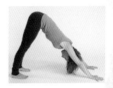

8 Downward Dog (p. 64)

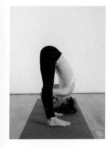

9 Forward Bend, Feet Wide (p. 62)

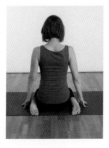

10 Reclining Hero (p. 98)

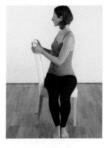

11 Bharadvajasana I (p. 94)

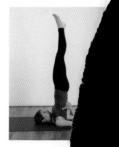

12 Shoulder (p. 120)

13 Plough (p. 122); 14 Seated Forward Bend (p. 70);
15 Corpse (p. 129); (not shown).

Session 2

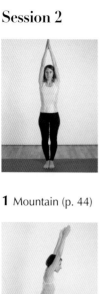

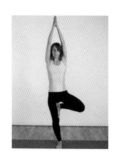

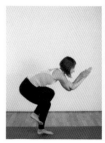

1 Mountain (p. 44) **2** Cow's Head (p. 74) **3** Tree (p. 48) **4** Eagle (p. 50)

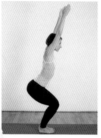

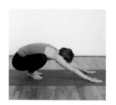

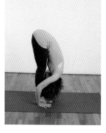

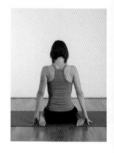

5 The Chair (p. 46) **6** Garland (p. 88) **7** Standing Forward Bend (p. 62) **8** Hero (p. 72)

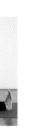

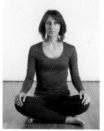

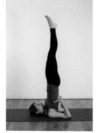

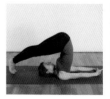

p. 68) **10** Easy Cross-Legged Pose (p. 78) **11** Shoulder Stand (p. 120) **12** Plough (p. 122)

13 Head-to-Knee Bend (p. 84); 14 One-Leg- Forward Bend (p. 86); 15 Maricy's Pose I (p. 90); 16 Seated Forward Bend (p. 70) 17 Reclining Twist (p. 114); I8 Corpse (p. 129) (not shown).

Session 3

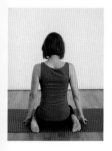

1 Hero (p. 72)

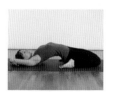

2 Reclining Hero (p. 98)

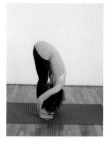

3 Standing Forward Bend (p. 62)

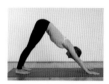

4 Dog (p. 64)

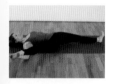

5 Leg Stretching (p. 108)

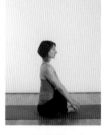

6 Tailor (p. 80)

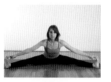

7 Seated Angle Pose (p. 82)

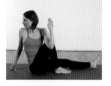

8 Maricy's Pose III (p. 92)

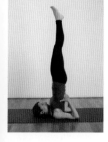

9 Shoulder Stand (p. 120)

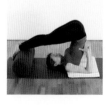

10 Supported Plough (p. 122)

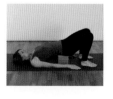

11 Bridge (p. 112)

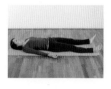

12 Corpse (p. 129)

Index